What Is Healing?

Awaken Your
Intuitive Power for
Health and Happiness

Catherine Carrigan

What Is Healing? Awaken Your Intuitive Power
for Health and Happiness

Edited and formatted by:
Launchpad Press, Cody, WY
www.launchpad-press.com

Disclaimer: This book does not dispense medical advice. The health information in this book is of a general nature and cannot substitute for the advice of a medical professional (your medical doctor, registered nurse, or pharmacist). Nothing in this book should be construed as an attempt to offer a medical opinion or otherwise engage in the practice of medicine. The information in this book is not intended to be a substitute for consulting with your medical professional about your specific health condition. Please see your medical professional about any specific questions you have about your personal health.

ISBN-13: 978-1-62747-0025

Printed in the United States of America

CONTENTS

INTRODUCTION

"It is love alone that leads to right action. What
brings order in the world is to love and let love do
what it will. "

—JIDDU KRISHNAMURTI

What is healing? Is it merely a physical
transformation, such as when you stop blowing your
nose or coughing after the typical seven days to a
week that you suffer through a cold? Is it a whole
body experience, such as the subtle integration
that occurs in the relaxation at the conclusion of a
yoga practice? Is it a sense of relief in your mind,
like when you shut your eyes to meditate, the world
drawing inward, stilling your senses momentarily?
Is healing what actually happens when you get the
test results back from your doctor that say, "Cancer
Free," the imprimatur of official health listed in detail
in the laboratory report numbers? It is my belief and
experience that true healing is all of this and more.

I am a professional health intuitive and holistic healer. I have written this book to share my journey and inspire you on yours. I could have written this book in cookbook fashion: first chop wood, then boil water, and then peel the potatoes. But it's my experience that true healing is not a linear process. It has scenic detours, dead ends, surprise vistas, and is something that is always unfolding.

I am blessed to have both an outdoor and indoor garden. Outdoors, I raise herbs, annuals and perennials, vegetables for juicing, bulbs, roses, shrubs, trees, and vines. Indoors, I primarily raise orchids, though I also enjoy a bonsai tree on my desk and a little Douglas fir that I bought one year at Target that has grown taller every year in my living room.

The process of fostering the growth of another living being—either plant or human—is a delight for the soul. Plants go through seven stages:

- Pollination
- Fertilization
- Seed formation
- Seed dispersal
- Germination
- Growth
- Flowering and pollination, allowing the cycle to continue.

Many of the major stages of growth seem to be invisible to the naked eye. There are times in my garden where nothing seems to be happening. For example, I planted a perennial orchid last year in the bed just outside my studio. It was flowering purple petals when I put it in the ground, but soon the blossom faded, then the roots and stems and leaves faded. It seemed to be gone completely, but I drove a stake in the ground where I had placed it, being careful not to disturb the soil around it.

I waited and then I watched. I would go out and look at the area around the stake.

At last, it is putting out three new shoots and seems to have tripled in size just in the process of resting through the winter!

Indoors, my orchids may sit for months in an apparent state of quiescence. Then one day, I go down to my studio and a bud has formed. Days later, the bud splits into two, a drop of sticky liquid appearing at the end. My excitement builds. I turn the pot toward the sun and wait. In its own good time, the bud opens, and then a true dance begins. The petals rotate, lifting their heads, turning until the entire blossom opens. After a time, the colors begin to fade slightly. Then one day they turn brown and droop and fall away.

So it is with people. We go through major stages of growth. Birth. Our first day of kindergarten, the first day at school, our first love. Off to college. First job. Marriage. Birth of our own children. Second job, third job, another career. Aging of our parents. Our children leave home. Death of our parents. Our own aging. Loss of our partner. Our own death. Our legacy living on through our children, through our work and all that we have built, contributed, and given away throughout our lifetime.

It may take years of preparation for each

transition. We may not even be ready for any of these transitions but they happen to us anyway, just in the due course of being human. We can resist the changes, or we can learn to love ourselves through every part of the process, yielding and allowing, knowing that the force that opened our embryo is still guiding us through every part of the process all the way to the end.

I notice that my clients may go through major changes. I may help them get well, overcome an illness, a loss, a job transition, or a life transition. Then they may go away for years at a time, only to reappear on my doorstep at the next step of their lives, just like the perennial orchid that seemed to disappear, only to push through the soil at a greater stage of evolution.

I share my personal stories in hopes of giving you a glimpse of the way I think when I look at a person's body, when I talk to a client, or proceed with a healing.

If I were going to read a book about how to make money, for example, I could read a list of rules or guidelines from someone who has found success for himself or herself by following these rules. However, I would find the story a lot more compelling if I knew the man telling me how to make a fortune had grown up living out of trailer someplace before he made his mark. Now that would be a man I might listen to quite carefully.

Despite my career as a health professional, I wasn't always very healthy myself.

The list of ailments—mental, physical, and

spiritual—that I have overcome in my life is so long that I have oftentimes said the prayer, "Dear God, I promise, next time I will just read about it in a book!"

At the time of this writing, I am 53 years old. During the course of my life, I have overcome:

- Chronic earaches, colds, and flus as a child
- Crooked teeth that required braces, a nightguard and eventually several biteguards
- Anorexia nervosa as a teenager, where I got down to ninety pounds
- Bulimia
- Loss of my menstrual cycle for years at a time (twice during my lifetime, both as a teenager and in my mid-thirties)
- Head injuries due to physical abuse as a child
- Physical abuse, both as a child and an adult, that caused me to join a YWCA support group for battered women for two years
- Spent one week in a mental hospital during my college years
- Got off lithium and antidepressants after eighteen years
- Chronic depression
- Severe hypoglycemia that would cause near fainting even while driving a car
- Chronic fatigue syndrome
- Addison's disease from severe adrenal burnout
- Panic attacks while riding in a car
- Parasites, including at least five different types of parasites
- Ulcers from *h. pylori*
- Severe food allergies

- Candida
- Hepatitis
- Lumps in my breasts
- Asthma so bad I lost my breath walking across a flat parking lot, requiring steroid inhalers
- Environmental allergies, so I had to receive injections twice a week for years
- Environmental sensitivities, so that I would get dizzy walking into a garden after it had been sprayed with chemicals or in a store that had fluorescent lights
- Severe pain in both feet
- Pain in my left knee
- Hip pain that resulted in limping (several times)
- Herniated disks in my lower back
- Shoulder pain from ripping tendons and ligaments in my right shoulder
- Broken fingers in both my hands
- Trigeminal neuralgia
- Hot flashes from menopause

Growing up the daughter of an opthalmologist, I was paraded to a wide variety of medical doctors, psychologists, and psychiatrists. I have great appreciation for all these well-meaning professionals. I was always a dutiful patient and did exactly what the doctors prescribed for me, as I sincerely wanted to feel better.

However, it was only when I began studying and practicing alternative healing methods that I began to experience mental and physical health on any appreciable level.

I have been truly healed by kinesiology, Reiki, yoga, tai chi, qi gong, nutritional supplements of all kinds (including herbs, vitamins and minerals, amino acids), juicing, healthy eating, meditation, flower essences, karmic clearing, quantum healing, craniosacral therapy, chiropractic, acupuncture and acupressure, far infrared saunas, colonics, resting, and journaling.

One of the healers who helped me, Sue Maes of Ontario, Canada, once said to me, "Most people who were as sick as you were would have just given up."

If you were to see me today, you might think, "Wow, what a healthy person!"

I didn't always know how to read the body, tease out transformation in others, or lead them to find their own light. In fact, I still question whether I actually know anything, and on many days I believe I probably don't really know anything at all.

But I have a guide that has helped me through my own healing process: I rely on my intuition. In sharing with you the stories in this book, my hope is that you will enjoy the journey and, in the process, awaken your own intuitive gifts of knowing, seeing, hearing, and feeling. You can learn to use your own intuitive powers to guide yourself toward greater health and happiness.

Please have fun as you read these words. In my view, if you are not having fun, what is the point, after all?

Catherine Carrigan
Atlanta, January 2013

PART I:

UNDERSTANDING THE NATURE OF INTUITION AND UNCONDITIONAL LOVE

Chapter 1. We Are Not Alone

"The intuitive mind is a sacred gift and the rational mind is a faithful servant. We have created a society that honors the servant and has forgotten the gift."

—Albert Einstein

The love and light of God shines equally upon us all. I notice it every day when I am in my studio. The windows are full of orchids. The room is filled with the aromas of essential oils, the loving presence of my rescue dog, Belle, and me. Together, Belle and I overlook a blue jar fountain, euphorbia and double-blossom apple begonias, and a park across the way that is full of hawks and owls—even a deer that one of my neighbors saw after coming home from a late night listening to music. But one of the most unique treasures I have encountered often while in my studio is the presence of angels; I have even photographed some of them and the space they leave, which is full of light.

Angels are all around us—everywhere and omnipresent. I consider them to be proof that God loves us, wants to protect us, and that He is always there.

The space an angel leaves may be full of light. I have photographed a portal outside my studio.

One night a few years ago a massive tornado blitzed through town. Earlier that day I had met with my gardener, Gabe Horrisberger, to discuss the massive tree that had been hanging diagonally over my home, from the front right corner to the back left corner. He and I had stood in my front yard looking worried and discussing what to do. I needed his advice, and asked to meet with him because I was concerned about what would happen if the tree fell on my roof. The next thing you know, I'm up all night praying, from maybe eleven p.m. on. The howling wind accelerated around midnight. By the next morning, trees were down all over the neighborhood.

My neighbors behind me had lost power—an outage that would last four days. There were trees on cars, trees on top of houses. One couple found their home split in two. But I was fine. My home had been completely protected. It later took five guys an entire day of work to cut that tree down.

A friend and I had scheduled to attend a class at Emory University the next morning. There were so many trees blocking the streets all over the city that it took us an hour to pick our way through the maze. When we finally arrived at the campus, we couldn't get in because we were completely blocked, not by the lines of traffic going nowhere but by the trees that prevented anyone from crossing.

A few days later, I went for a walk in my neighborhood carrying my iPhone so that I could listen to tunes. When I arrived home, I started snapping photographs. And then I saw it: a shield of light. It was so remarkable I photographed the light cluster multiple times to make sure it was not just a camera mistake. From then on, the angels would show up in my photographs, completely unbidden and occurring at unexpected times. (You can see some of these photographs on my website, *www.catherinecarrigan.com.*)

One day my very excellent painter came to stain my back deck. It was a glorious spring day. The air was full of light. I brought out my iPhone and started taking pictures of my garden, the flowers around the fountain, and my deck. I was walking toward the front of my home when I saw Belle by the front door. I snapped a picture of her by the door and turned away. And there they were again, the angels! I could see them immediately in the photograph. I had taken pictures of fuzzy light by my door before but, this time, I could see their faces, heads, and wings.

All of this occurred on a glorious, sunny day in Atlanta, even though, simultaneously, halfway around the world, a tsunami had hit Japan, disabling a nuclear reactor there.

A few days later, I had conducted a medical intuitive reading with a woman in Tokyo. I had met her the year before at a tai chi retreat in Sedona, Arizona. I had heard from my tai chi friends that she was in distress; I reached out to her. I told her to get out of Tokyo immediately, because it had already been affected by radiation. She did not believe me initially, because the authorities had not yet confirmed what we now know: there was a major radiation leak at the Fukushima Daiichi Nuclear Power Plant, less than 200 miles away. I even encouraged her to leave for America if she could.

She was nervous and doubtful; she surfed the internet constantly before packing up her belongings and her two cats and heading off to southern Japan for a distant relative's house. I continued to communicate with her and also reached out to my healer friend, Don Dennis, in Scotland. I asked him if he knew of any remedies for nuclear radiation exposure. He didn't, so he created a flower essence to balance the effects of radiation called Energy Matrix, which included seawater, so the remedy could pass the inspectors and be distributed into Japan.

Both Don and I recognized the magnitude of the situation, and he immediately shipped off a few bottles of his new remedy to the woman hovering in a relative's bedroom somewhere in southern Japan.

There she was, gluten intolerant, eating food that didn't agree with her, out of her comfort zone, living with two cats in a single room. But she was not alone. One of the biggest myths that causes us to suffer as human beings is the belief that we are alone. However, I believe that God is all there is. I believe that it's all one energy, and that one energy is actually God.

If it is all God, I therefore reason that it's all good.

And because everything that exists—the rocks, the stars, the orchids in my studio, you, me—is part of that one energy, that means we are all connected.

Sometimes people ask me how I know what I know. I just laugh, because the truth is I have just learned how to use my gift. Only after I learned how to use my gift have I begun to understand logically how it is and why it is that this might actually work. Because we are all connected at the molecular level, at the cellular level, at the energy level, at the divine level, everything is everywhere knowable all the time if we just learn how to tune into it.

We may feel alone—I have felt intensely lonely at many times in my own life and have often prayed and asked for guidance about how to release the sharp pain of this feeling—but that feeling is just exactly that, a pain, but not actually the larger truth.

Sitting in my home in Atlanta, I could focus my intuitive mind and read exactly what was going on not only with this dear lady in Tokyo but also with the bigger picture, which was that she and everybody else there was in danger of the radiation from the accident at the nuclear plant. I was able to do that because I have set my intention to serve God for the highest good, and when communicating with others, I ask Spirit that I be shown what it is they need to know in any given moment.

I have learned to trust what comes through me, laughing at times at what I am told, as when it first comes out of my mouth it sometimes seems a bit odd even to me until I too understand the bigger picture. I thought it was no coincidence that I literally saw the angels by my front door that day. In my mind, everything has vibration and angels are spiritual beings of such a high frequency they go beyond the energy any of us mere human beings can ever hold in our life of the flesh.

Somehow, I must have needed to be lifted up and comforted by the presence of angels around my home just as I was attempting to ease the mind of the lady in Tokyo sitting by her computer, searching for news, trying to understand what she should do and where she should go.

I understood how it feels to be lonely, to feel lost, afraid, and without guidance, but I wanted the lady in Tokyo to know that even though she might be feeling that way, in fact she was loved and being looked after in a very careful way.

CHAPTER 2. THE FIELD OF UNCONDITIONAL LOVE

"To understand the nature of God, it is necessary only to know the nature of love itself. To truly know love is to know and understand God; and to know God is to understand love."

—DAVID HAWKINS, M.D.

There is a field of unconditional love that surrounds all of us. Some people call this field God. Most people recognize God, Universal Source, Divinity, or their Higher Power, even if they don't understand the field. The field cannot be seen, measured, quantified, or touched, but it is the most powerful force in the entire universe.

This field has its own intelligence. It is all-knowing but beyond intellect. Those who try to measure with only their rational, left-brained mind cannot fully comprehend its magnitude.

It's important for all of us to know the thoughts of

God. All else is mere smoke and mirrors, illusions. And this field, God has all the information we will ever need—all the guidance and all our answers. If we can access this field that we all call God, we simply get a bigger picture. From this larger perspective we can make more informed choices for the highest good of all.

If I know just one-tenth of what is going on, I may or may not be able to make good decisions. But if I have even more information, from all different angles—the macro and the micro—my ability to act for the highest good will most probably be greater.

Many people pray every day to raise their level of consciousness. Some even ask to be enlightened. In my mind, this is asking to see all that is from this bigger perspective—quite literally, to be more conscious of all that is.

In a way, asking for this, praying about this, and setting your intention for enlightenment is almost asking for trouble unless you are also quite serious about serving God, this global consciousness. It takes serious courage on your part to ask for this bigger picture, because you may discover that what you know, hear, feel, or see is in direct contradiction to how things first appeared to you.

When you feel more of what is going on, you feel what other people are feeling. This could be good, bad, or indifferent. You could feel other people's pain and other people's suffering. You could put your hands on someone and feel the intensity of their ache. You could feel the cars that drive by your house.

One of my friends who is quite sensitive felt the

trauma the day a gunman shot dead twenty-seven children and adults in Newton, Connecticut, even before she heard the actual news. She spent the rest of the day visiting two different healers because of the intense shock that rippled through her entire body.

When you hear more of what is going on, you can indeed hear the whispers of angels and you can hear your own guardian angel speaking to you. One of my clients, the top salesperson in her company, said it this way: "After ten minutes, I know not only what other people are saying, I hear what they aren't saying." That might make you another top salesperson. But you could also hear other people's disappointment or that they don't really like you or what you are selling.

When you see and know more of what is going on, you may also know that other people aren't quite ready to have all the information—not just yet. When you are more conscious, you then have to be more responsible with the insights you receive.

How could I, living in Atlanta with my dog, worrying about what paint color to put on the walls of my office (I must have considered twenty different shades of grey), paying to have my porch stained that glorious day in March, know what was going on with a woman in Japan I had met only once?

The answer is quite simple: unconditional love. Many people try to access their intuition, knowing that intuitive gifts offer us something quite special, but they go about it in a left-brain way without acknowledging that intuition actually is an integral part of what we have always been as a species.

What is intuition? Although others may have contributed their own understanding, I will humbly attempt to describe intuition through my own limited experience through using my gifts and teaching other people how to access theirs.

Intuition is the gift of knowing, hearing, feeling, or seeing through our spiritual senses. Just as we are blessed with a brain through which we learn and understand, ears with which to hear, fingers and toes and a body through which to feel, and a pair of eyes through which we learn to see, I believe our soul is also blessed with senses.

This is why, in my way of thinking, people who have reported near-death experiences are able to describe in great detail their hospital room and also what other people are thinking, feeling, or saying. And this is also why, if we shut our eyes, we may still be able to see a picture of what is going on; why, if we are miles away or alone in dead silence, we can still hear a voice speaking to us; and why, when we are continents away, we can know the facts about another human being in need.

Just as the brain has its own way of operating, the ears another, the eyes yet another, and the body, fingers and toes yet another means, our intuition can be further divided into separate skills.

There is the gift of psychic knowing, also called claircognizance. When you use this gift, you just know stuff—even if you don't have any idea how you know it. There is also clairaudience, clairsentience, and clairvoyance. I will be discussing each of these gifts in further detail later on in the book.

Each of the gifts works in slightly different ways, but when you are using your intuition in practicality, more than likely you will learn to use a little bit of all your gifts.

For example, when I am having a conversation in person with my great friend Virginia Wright, I may be listening to her, watching her facial expressions, feeling the emotions behind her words and remembering our past history together.

So it is when we use intuition. I may see a picture or symbol, just know stuff, feel an emotion or a body sensation or hear words or information. In other words, it all works together, and only in retrospect do we piece apart what we just knew, what we saw, what we heard and what we felt.

If you think about the Aboriginals in Australia and other early communities of mankind, native man has always used intuition as a means not just of communication but also of actual navigation, of finding the way.

Here is a thought you may not have considered before: intuition is a byproduct of unconditional love. When we allow ourselves to experience unconditional love in our lives, what we are able to know, see, feel, hear, and access is actually unlimited, unbounded by time. You can know whatever it is that you need to know about anyone or anything or at any time, past or present, as long as you love unconditionally.

Since most of us have only given or received love in a conditioned or partial way, the idea that anyone or anything can be read like an open book may seem foreign or scary—or even fantastical and ridiculous, absurd and fallacious. The truth is you can learn to love unconditionally and, in the process, open up your own intuition to heights you may never before have deemed imaginable.

What is unconditional love? I believe that unconditional love is both a noun, a verb, and a way of being.

Let's talk first about what it's not. Unconditional love is not the high you get when you first fall in love with a man or a woman, however insanely delicious and delightful that experience may be. That is something passed down from our cave man and cave woman selves. Instinctual, driven by hormones, inherent in our species, fun, full of ups and downs, dramas and disappointments, the stuff of every country music song and half the other songs ever written: that's still not unconditional love.

Unconditional love is a gift of the heart. It's a gift that we can both give and receive that comes with no strings attached, no qualifications, reservations, footnotes, asterisks, objections, judgments, or other kinds of fine print legalese that later have to be uncovered, argued over, or cried about.

To love another unconditionally is for your soul to love another soul. It's an all-encompassing way of loving another that may give full value to all the other person's faults, failings, and foibles and, at the same time, being fully aware of all of that, to overlook the lot completely, and be able to grasp his or her divine essence. It's a way of loving that goes beyond all time and cannot be broken or stopped based on circumstances. Unconditional love as a way of being means, to me, to fully embrace another person, from your heart to his or her heart, with complete acceptance.

When I was in college, a friend of mine who had never even had the privilege of completing high school, Eula Mae Brown, used to write me the most touching letters.

She wrote by hand, so I had to struggle over every word, reading each line several times just to grasp her meaning. Even though it was difficult for me to make out what she said many times, she ended every letter with a line that would take my breath away: "Take all mistakes for love."

Eula Mae was a person who spent much of her life in prayer. She knew instinctively that although she had suffered the loss of one of her daughters, who had been accidentally shot when a neighbor was cleaning his gun, that all things come from God and, therefore, it is all good. There was no mistake that was actually a mistake, she was saying at the end of her letters. It's all the unconditional love of God.

This is a book about intuition, for sure. But it is also a book about how you can access unconditional love—which, at the end of the day, is what we are all aching for at very deep levels.

When I think of people living in rubble heaps in India, or people whom I have never met in China or Australia, what overwhelms me is the sense that we are all connected. We are all one species, for sure, but that species is directed and connected by this field of unconditional love.

We breathe in, we breathe out. We inhale and exhale the same molecules. We are natural recyclers of the same energy, whether or not we realize it. My goal in this book is to teach you how to access unconditional love in your life and, in so doing, open up your intuition—available to you so long as you learn how to love deeply and with your whole heart.

CHAPTER 3. SCENES OF UNCONDITIONAL LOVE

"Cease trying to work everything out with your minds. It will get you nowhere. Live by intuition and inspiration and let your whole life be Revelation."

—EILEEN CADDY

I was visiting my family down in Savannah, Georgia, one weekend. I have never found my visits to be enjoyable: my parents had long since divorced and remarried, and it was always awkward for me to go back and forth, as if I were an ambassador trying to renegotiate the Mason-Dixon line shortly after the War between the States.

Going down to Savannah always became a matter of whom to visit first and then checking all the boxes: (1) Go to visit my father across the river in South Carolina; (2) go visit my mother downtown; and, (3) hopefully, make it out to the south side of town to visit my grandparents, who were basically bedridden in a nursing home.

I remember trying to think of things that would please my grandmother. At that point, one of her few remaining pleasures was sweets, so she would gobble the candies I bought her at Walmart. I sent her a teddy bear as I intuitively felt she needed to hug something or someone; my grandfather was across the hall in the nursing home in a room of his own. My grandparents had been married for well over sixty years.

When I finally came to visit after sending her the teddy bear, I was so sad to see it sitting on her dresser, staring at her in the bed, her eyes shut, flesh hanging off her thin, frail bones. I wanted to hug the bear myself as I sat next to her on our brief visits. There seemed so little to say. She could hold my hand, but not much else.

My grandmother and I had always been very close. I looked like her and she looked like me. When I was younger, we would kid around with each other about who was taller. We would line up, back to back, and we would discover that we were both the same height, both petite women. It wasn't much to have in common, but we probably shared a sense of insignificance in a world dominated by the men in our lives.

My grandfather was a kindly scientist. Even after he retired, he continued to invent contraptions of all kinds. My grandmother surrounded their home with antiques. My grandfather surrounded the garden with camellias, and he created one that he named after my grandmother and one he named after me.

We all loved each other very much and had been greatly saddened by the divorce of my parents.

So, on that fateful Sunday, I had gone to church with my father. It was a country church with plain wooden benches and a stained pine floor. For some reason, as I was sitting in church, about an hour away from Savannah, I began crying uncontrollably. I had experienced a few times in my life when tears overwhelmed me, but this felt different. I had no idea why I had been crying so much. I just could not stop crying. I wept so bitterly that the floor underneath my feet became wet with tears.

Terribly embarrassed to be crying so much in the middle of a boring church service, I resolved to return to Atlanta at once. At the end of the service, I said good-bye to my father and headed back to my home.

When I got to my house, I received a telephone call. My grandmother had just died. Suddenly, my overwhelming sense of uncontrollable grief made sense. Even though I had no idea what was happening, I had picked up on her passing.

Paradoxically, as I had been trying to visit everyone during that trip, I had spent time with my mother downtown and that Sunday morning had driven all the way to Tillman, South Carolina, to visit my father, so there had been no time to see my grandparents in the nursing home. I knew they needed me much more than either my mother or father, but I did not have a moment to make the drive out to see them. And, as I got the call, I realized why.

I would never have left my grandmother's side. I

am not sure I could have ever let her go, nor would she have allowed herself to pass if I had been with her. She needed to be away from me in order to give herself permission to pass at last.

In my immediate grief, I opened my journal. I took out a pen and began writing. Suddenly, I heard her voice, and there she was.

"I love you more than life itself," she told me.

"Don't leave me!" I replied, writing the words between my tears.

"Don't worry," she said to me. "I will be in your writing."

Some of us have been lucky enough to experience a love of this depth. I had needed my grandparents through my difficult childhood. My parents did their best, I am sure, but it was with my grandparents that I experienced the feeling of unconditional love—not that I could do no wrong, but that no matter what wrong I did I would eventually be forgiven. With them I was treasured; I was precious.

I remember my grandmother tucking me into bed at night, telling me all the while how much she loved me. This is unconditional love.

Paradoxically, it was my grandmother who first spoke to me of anything metaphysical. She talked to me about hypnosis as she swung a watch in front of my eyes. She also told me about the poem she wrote and published about getting engaged to my grandfather. I didn't quite take it all in, but I understood and appreciated her interests.

Chapter 4. My Professor

"What we are communicates far more eloquently than anything we say or do."

—Stephen Covey

When I arrived at Brown University, Kermit Champa was my professor for Art History 101. I wasn't sure what I wanted to study, and in fact wasn't sure about just about anything.

I had made the mistake of showing up for college with a wardrobe of skirts when practically every other female wore blue jeans. I had a little plaid skirt that I wore to Professor Champa's lectures. I was one of literally hundreds of students in that lecture hall, so I doubted if he knew who I was at first.

I was so sure that someone would discover that I was actually stupid and that it was a mistake for Brown University to have accepted me. I felt like an imposter, so I studied very hard. This fear of inadequacy made me quite nervous. I had trouble breathing and had a lot of allergies and stomach problems. I would be at the library often when it first opened for the day, subscribing to a very strict discipline and hoping not to get kicked out when someone finally discovered me for being who I thought I was: stupid and worthless.

After handing in one of the papers I had written that year, Professor Champa asked for me to meet him his office. *At last,* I thought, *I have been discovered!* It was true: someone had figured out how stupid I was and I was about to go down for my talking to. I remember being quite shaky as I showed up at his office. I was on the verge of tears.

As fate would have it, Professor Champa didn't tell me that I was stupid. He said I had written the most brilliant undergraduate art history paper he had ever read! Professor Champa and I would go on to be quite close. We spoke nearly every week for twenty-seven years.

Being so young at the time, I did not realize what a huge gift he had given me. But now I do. I would call him through all phases and directions of my life: in love, feeling lost, wanting an answer to a question I knew he would have the wisdom to share. This was unconditional love.

It was only in later years, as an adult, that I realized how kind he had been to be the father I always wanted but never had. I loved him back, as many students did. He kept his boundaries, but he kept encouraging me. He applauded me when I went for an unconventional career.

"I am proud of you," he said to me. "You did not

just go for the money."

About a year before he died, I received a psychic message that my father was about to pass away.

Oh well, I thought. My real father and I were not close. He had never been a support to me in the way I really needed it. I had spent two years in a support group for battered women before understanding what kind of relationship my true father and I had actually had. Through years of inner work, I had come to an acceptance of it all, but I turned to Professor Champa when I really wanted guidance and support.

Shortly after I received this message, I found out that Professor Champa had contracted pneumonia. When I called him on the phone, and he told me about his condition, I said to him, "People don't just get pneumonia."

I recommended that he go get thoroughly checked out by a medical doctor. Within days, he was diagnosed with lung cancer. I immediately went into grieving; I had already seen the end result. I offered to come up and live with him—take care of him, make him fresh juice, and do healing work with him—but he declined.

The last time I actually spoke to him was a few days before my birthday. But his spirit came to me, and his soul asked me to take care of his widow, Judith.

"Of course!" I said. Professor Champa had guided and protected me for twenty-seven years before he passed away in 2004. I immediately began calling his widow. I put her in my will. She went through years of hell, losing a husband, a cat, then her father, then her job. But I made sure I was there for her as Professor Champa had been for me. That is unconditional love.

CHAPTER 5. SOUL MATES

"If you judge people, you have no time to love them."

—MOTHER THERESA

I was married for many years to a man I thought I was very happy with. Then one day a gentleman named Ken and his wife showed up at one of the qi gong classes I was teaching. I had received guidance years before that it was very important for me to teach qi gong. I thought at the time that it was all about the energy, as qi gong is an energy exercise and clears and balances your energy field.

I taught the class every Wednesday afternoon at five-thirty p.m. I figured it was the perfect time of the week to do it: it was Hump Day, and everybody who needed more energy to get through the rest of the week could simply join me in the garden where we could enjoy all five elements: the sun, the earth—from the blue jar fountain around which we practiced—the fresh air, the water from the flowing fountain itself. And, to top it off, there were all of the flowers, trees, and shrubs in my beautiful garden. Teaching qi gong fed my soul.

My class had never gotten very big, but I never minded it. It was important for me to teach qi gong, I knew, so I kept doing it, even if only one person showed up to join me. When Ken and his wife showed up they had been to Sedona, Arizona, attending a lecture by Dr. David Hawkins, author of *Power vs. Force* (Hay House, 1995), my favorite book of all time. While they were there, they heard about qi gong and decided they wanted to find an instructor in Atlanta.

The three of us immediately hit it off, and they began attending my class. Eventually, we joined with others to form a spiritual book club. We met together to read Dr. Hawkins and other spiritual authors. The group became very important to all of us.

Six months later, Ken was the only person to show up for one of my classes. Because it was just the two of us, he spoke to me frankly and privately. He told me that he had fallen in love with me! He felt his feelings for me were wrong and he was looking for a way to make them disappear.

I had hoped that I would appear very ugly to him. I am sure I had turned quite pale. I protested mightily. I understood where he was coming from, and I did not think badly of him. I knew how these things could just happen. Like Ken, I was in a committed relationship; I had been praying every night to be a good wife to my husband. It was very important to me to stay married to my husband. I worked out of my home, I loved my home and my work, and I wanted to keep my status quo.

Ken suffered much. He stayed away. He and his wife went to marriage counseling. He did everything he could to forget about me. He cut the cords between us in every way he could think of. The feelings were not only immovable but they kept growing. From time to time he would call me on the phone to tell me he loved me, and I would discourage him from going any further. I am not usually mean, but I was actually mean to him.

Then, finally, after two and a half years of this, Ken called me again. He had been praying that if I was not his soul mate, that God would send him the person who actually was.

"I love you," Ken said to me.

I had heard that before, so I was not impressed or distracted from my original position. But this time he added, "And I know you love me, too. Face it!" Ever the turtle in these matters, I continued to protest.

I remember sitting in my office on the phone with him, completely bewildered, stubborn, and insistent. About a week later, I realized that he was right: I loved him also. It was probably the most challenging spiritual insight I have ever had.

What is a spiritual person to do: stay married to someone you now know you no longer love, or go out on a limb like a complete idiot to be with someone your soul is telling you that you *have to* be with?

I am not a cruel person, or at least I don't think so.

In the past, when Ken had talked to me, I could not bear the thought of hurting my husband or his wife. In the end, both Ken and I chose to be together. We went through two and a half of the hardest years of our lives to free ourselves. But now we are together.

"I love you more than I have ever loved anyone," Ken has said to me. "I love you now. I will always love you."

I had not been looking for him, and he had not been looking for me. But there we were. Somehow, in all the inner work we had done up until that point in our lives, we had opened ourselves to let more love in. And then we found each other.

I have learned over the years to be careful what I ask for. Sometimes we pray, with deep sincerity and from the great depths of our heart, "Dear God, please help me grow spiritually." When we say this prayer, with all honesty, we may end up having to face ourselves—our shortcomings and our current challenges—more squarely than we had thought ourselves ready for.

I was quite shocked that this situation manifested in my life because, like many people, I had been ignoring and even fighting my own intuitive guidance about it. I just refused to allow myself to go there. My left-brained mind had a certain order that I thought I needed in my life, and I was determined to keep things the way they were.

In order to access our intuition, however, we must be *neutral*. As one of my many teachers explained once, one way to understand neutral is to ask yourself questions the answers to which you really don't care about. How many tiles are in your home? How many cans of paint did it take to cover the walls of your room? Who cares!

It's easy to be neutral when we are not emotionally involved in the answer. When you are in neutral, you are completely open to whatever information needs to come through at that time for the highest good. We simply can't be neutral if our emotions get in the way.

That is why it's important, when we truly want to access our intuition, to do emotional clearing work on an ongoing basis so that we don't accumulate a backlog of repressed emotions that are clouding our guidance.

And we also can't be neutral if we are resistant. Resistance is a normal, natural part of being human. Most of us are more comfortable with what we know, no matter how chaotic or wrong it actually happens to be for us. As Neale Donald Walsh says, "Life begins at the end of your comfort zone." It takes great courage to face our resistance and look at the truth. In this case, when I went into acceptance I was able to open myself to unconditional love.

Chapter 6. Belle

"The commonest kinds of seemingly telepathic response are the anticipation by dogs and cats of their owners coming home; the anticipation of owners going away; the anticipation of being fed; cats disappearing when their owners intend to take them to the vet; dogs knowing when their owners are planning to take them for a walk; and animals that get excited when their owner is on the telephone, even before the telephone is answered."

—Rupert Sheldrake

I joke nowadays about how my life can be seen in terms of B.B. and A.B.: before Belle and after Belle. For most of my life, in B.B. time, I had been a cat person, specifically a fat orange cat person. I had grown up with both dogs and cats in the house, but the dogs I grew up with were all hunting dogs and had not been close or really all that connected to me.

I had a succession of fat orange cats that miraculously seemed to blow up to prize-winning sizes without me doing much of anything extra. I seemed to think that I was content to have just an orange cat when a business associate of mine at the time told me about a little dog he had seen at the Atlanta Pet Rescue.

At first, I saw her picture online on the organization's website. Belle was brown and white and fluffy with long curly ears. The website seemed to me almost like a dating website, with each pet's photograph and a description about why each one was so special. I didn't dare go down and visit Belle in person, so my business associate and I became her guardian angels.

It's possible to be a dog's guardian angel simply by donating a certain amount of money that will be designated to help it get all the medical care and food and other requirements necessary for survival. But there is something to be said about adopting an animal, inviting it into your home, and providing unconditional love.

That is how I felt about Belle. I was proud to be Belle's guardian angel by providing monetary assistance for her care. It felt like I was doing something good, not just for Belle but also for the entire community. Then one day my business associate and I went to the pet rescue and I met her in person.

The first time I laid eyes on her, she was even more beautiful than she had appeared in her website picture, and was obviously very sensitive. She was also heavily depressed; when I saw her I wondered if she could ever keep up with me if we were to go for a walk. She seemed to mope around while all the other doggies in her kennel were playing happily. The volunteers at the pet rescue picked her up and took her into a special cage to meet me.

She sat in my lap. I hardly knew what to do, holding a dog for the first time in decades. She was very soft to the touch, and her softness seemed to extend not just to the fluffiness of her fur but deep inside her. And then she licked me! That was it. And the rest, as they say, is history.

We took Belle home and she became even softer. The whites at the edge of her eyes went away and she looked relaxed. She walked into the house and my orange cat Munchkin ignored her—*a good sign*, I thought.

I remember holding her and intuiting just how sad she was. Her eyes were bulging. Her skin was covered from head to toe with a horrible rash. When I took her to the vet, her ears were infected so badly they recommended an immediate ear operation and warned me that she might be deaf.

I don't have anything against operations when needed, but Belle had such severe panic attacks when I left her that I was afraid she would not be able to handle the separation anxiety of being found once again in a pen—I had learned that she had been placed with two pet rescue organizations. I didn't want her to wake up in a cage and wonder if she had been abandoned once again. So I turned to natural methods.

I treated her with flower essences. I used Reiki, a Japanese technique designed to reduce stress and promote healing, to treat her ears. I took her to a friend who does craniosacral therapy so I could lie on the table and hold her while she was being treated.

Eventually, Belle began to show signs of improvement. She learned how to walk on a leash and overcome her fear of walking in the neighborhood. At first I wanted her to stay upstairs when I went down to my studio to work, but Belle would have none of that. If I left her upstairs, she would immediately start crying. She had trained me.

Belle became part of my team when I did healing work; she sought permission to get on the table, greeted clients when they came in the door, and gave everyone the same amount of love and attention she had received when she became my dog.

Now Belle goes virtually everywhere possible with me—not just to work, but also to the bank, the UPS Store, the chiropractor, when I receive my own healing sessions, and when I go on a trip. She obviously views this as a natural order of things. Of course, she can't come to the grocery store, out to a restaurant, or to a movie. She can't come to yoga retreats or all the vacations I try to take. But she lets me know she is mine and we are a pair. Belle's softness warms the hearts of everyone who meets her.

Even the groomer told me, "I think she is the sweetest dog I have ever taken care of." Belle knows what it is like to have lost love and then rediscovered it. This is unconditional love.

Even the dog trainer said to me, "Most dogs are just out for themselves. Belle really loves you." It is hard to put my finger on exactly why Belle is such a lovable dog. Most pet owners are quite certain that their animal babies are the best, and I am just as prejudiced as anyone when it comes to my dog.

However, I can attest to the fact that Belle is adored by young and old, big kids and little babies, other dogs and even cats. Once, I brought little Belle over to play with her best friend, Kiwi, a yellow lab, while I was out teaching a yoga class. I had just arrived to roll out my yoga mat when I got a call on my cell phone. "We have your dog," the voice said.

Even though I had left Belle with dog cookies and her best friend, it had taken her no time at all to crawl under the fence and break away to freedom. Kiwi's owner, my friend Virginia Wright, headed home to sort out the situation. When she arrived, Virginia found Belle holding court in her front yard with a small group of eighth-grade girls, who were oohing and ahhing over her.

"They never act that way about Kiwi," Virginia observed.

Belle has four fluffy white paws, brown hair and ears, and at full fluff looks exactly like a little teddy bear. She allows virtually anyone to pick her up and hug her, which always appears to be a win-win situation, as the huggers feel comforted and little Belle seems to accept that being hugged is part of her job description.

Little children are instinctively drawn to her as she must appear to be a live version of the stuffed animals they collect at home.

Belle, Kiwi, Virginia, and I were in the Watkinsville, Georgia, Christmas parade in 2012. Belle sat in my lap and wore a little pointy red Christmas hat and allowed me to wave her paws at the passing crowd. As we were riding our float past the main announcer, he said, "Here are the ladies of Ashford Farm and their beautiful dogs!"

My painter, Dan Stone, has reported to me that he and his workers always know when I am on the way home because little Belle will start crying about four minutes before I actually arrive.

As I work from home and don't have any sort of regular schedule, this suggests to me that Belle has an intuitive connection with me that Rupert Sheldrake and others have reported in books such as *Dogs That Know When Their Owners Are Coming Home* (Broadway, 2011).

Although owning a dog is not a requirement for being or becoming an intuitive person, I do believe that having a canine companion is a great blessing for all those who want to open intuitive gifts, precisely because dogs open our hearts even more so than cats or other pets and keep our hearts open in good times as well as in bad.

"I think dogs are the most amazing creatures; they give unconditional love. For me, they are the role model for being alive," Gilda Radner once said.

Even though I have done intuitive readings for other dogs, horses, cats, and even a goat, I have not done intuitive readings about Belle because I know I would not be able to be neutral. Just as in any relationship, I can tell easily enough when she is trying to push my buttons, such as when she wants me to feed her more cookies and I feel she has had enough.

Belle, on the other hand, uses her intuition to read me all the time—and not just about when I am on the way home. She hides when it's time for her bath and sulks in the living room before I reach for her ear medicine. It is great fun for me to try to outsmart her in this department. It seems we are evenly matched.

I very much enjoy doing intuitive readings on all sorts of animals and feel a great sense of compassion and obligation to them because, unlike human patients, they are not typically able to point out where they are in pain or what happened to get them into trouble.

To communicate intuitively to an animal, the simplest way to begin is to set your intention for your soul to communicate with the animal's soul. This is the very same way that I communicate with little babies. Usually the first thing an animal will start talking to me about is—big drum roll—food! This usually makes me laugh, although I understand as most of the time their rations tend to be quite repetitive or missing in the nutrients they actually need.

Chapter 7. The Kinds of Unconditional Love

"Learning how to love is the goal and the purpose of spiritual life—not learning how to develop psychic powers, not learning how to bow, chant, do yoga, or even meditate, but learning to love. Love is the truth. Love is the light."

—Lama Surya Das

Many of us have had some degree of love in our lives. When we think of loving relationships we might bring to mind a grandparent, a teacher, or a soul mate who shows up unexpectedly. We might think of a beloved pet who goes everywhere with us. Maybe you have had a lifelong friend. Maybe your mother or father is always there for you. Maybe it's your boss or your aunt or your yoga instructor. Maybe it's your drinking buddy, your golf friend, or your pen pal.

Unconditional love in any form is the greatest

gift life can ever give you. It can be an unplanned event, even if longed for. Before we can understand unconditional love, we must ask a very critical question: are we open to loving and being loved?

There are four Greek words that help us to grasp the kinds of healthy love that are available to us: *storge, philia, eros,* and *agape.*

Storge means "affection," and it has to do with motherly love and the care we extend to members of our family. C. S. Lewis in his book, *The Four Loves* (Harcourt Brace, 1960), describes *storge* as arising out of our inherent need for love (Need-Love). "We are born helpless," Lewis writes. "As soon as we are fully conscious we discover loneliness. We need others physically, emotionally, intellectually; we need them if we are to know anything, even ourselves."

In Chinese medicine, there are two acupuncture meridians having to do with the heart. One of these is called the heart meridian, the other is called the pericardium meridian, related to the protective sack around the heart. This pericardium meridian is also sometimes referred to as the heart constrictor or circulation-sex meridian.

On an emotional level, this pericardium meridian has to do with bonding, and our ability to feel accepted and connected just as we are. When this meridian is working well, our heart swells with joy and pleasure. When it is out of balance emotionally, we feel rejected or disconnected.

The first person we connect with is usually our mother, with whom we develop *storge*, this kind of affectionate, familial love.

Once we have experienced connection, acceptance and bonding within our family, we often next experience *philia,* or friendship love. Little boys and girls often have a best friend, a person to whom they open their hearts, with whom they share their secrets and bond, finding common interests and mutual pleasure.

As we mature, we can experience *eros,* or passionate love. This kind of love is a marriage of our human animal, with our behavior driven by hormones, as well as by our human spirit, which is driven by the need for deep connection with another individual. As we have sex with another person, we form invisible cord connections from the energy centers known as our chakras to another person's chakra centers. The more we connect to another through all our chakras—not just our sexual center—the deeper and more fulfilling our passionate relationships can be. In this way, through passionate connection, we can learn to bond with another person spiritually, sharing our vision of life, having mutual topics of conversation, loving deeply, empathetically feeling the other person's feelings, enjoying sex, and ultimately forming a home together.

Once we have connected with our mother and family members, friends, and loved ones, we begin to experience an expanded sense of love, *agape.* This ultimately helps us to feel bonded and deeply connected to all that is, all humanity, God, and universal energy.

Agape helps us to expand our sense of self and, at the same time, to find meaning for ourselves within this greater whole. One of the ways to be truly happy in this life is to discover meaning, which usually requires seeing a bigger picture and making a contribution to something larger than just ourselves.

Ironically, as we bond to this greater whole, we can discover how to love ourselves even more deeply. First, we see ourselves through the eyes of our mother and family. We look like them, they look like us. We discover our original sense of identity. Then we see ourselves through the lens of our friends. We share the same interests, play on the same teams, work toward the same goals. And then, through passionate bonding and forming a home with a passionate loved one, we create a new sense of our very own family. We break away from the original tribe, form a tribe of our own, and discover a new sense of identity.

As we begin to see that we are part of the larger whole, we sense that we are part of the family of man, and we discover commonality with all people everywhere. We realize that as we breathe in, we are breathing in air that someone else breathed out. We become a meaningful part of a meaningful whole.

I remember once discussing the idea of being famous with my friend Sue Maes. Sue said, "Go up in an airplane and look down. Then tell me how important it is to be well known!" Looking down at the mountains, the clouds, the waters and the earth, the idea seems slightly ridiculous.

Often, our viewpoint of ourselves becomes so narrow that we forget the enormity of the world and the vastness of time and space. By expanding our sense of bonding and connection to this larger picture, we can eventually lose our sense of aloneness and set our intention to serve God for the highest good of all.

It is then, when we have set our intention to align our will with God's will, feeling, believing, and knowing our loving connection with all that is, that we can open up our intuition to our full potential.

CHAPTER 8. YOUR HEART

"Don't let the noise of other's opinions drown out your own inner voice. And most important, have the courage to follow your heart and intuition. They somehow already know what you truly want to become. Everything else is secondary."

—STEVE JOBS

It is a rare person who has not had his or heart completely broken by the age of thirty. By the age of fifty, the average person has had his or her heart broken so many times that he or she could be permanently depressed for the rest of life.

What breaks our heart could be the death of a loved one, the loss of a relationship, a divorce, loss of a job, or any number of issues. Years ago, I remember working with one of my male clients to heal his back pain. What many people don't realize is that often our lower back acts like a circuit breaker. If your heart experiences an overwhelming amount of stress, often your lower back will give out to make you stop and rest to keep you from having a heart attack. This syndrome is called "cardiac low back" in alternative healing.

This gentleman had tried everything he could think of to heal his back, but was still experiencing excruciating pain. He often had trouble walking through his back yard, even though he was only in his mid-forties.

I used a combination of yoga, movement re-education for his muscles, and energy work to heal him, but the biggest shift came when we addressed the issues with his ex-wife.

Even though my client had been divorced for about twelve years, he was still energetically connected to his ex-wife. I could tell because I could count the cord connections at the chakra energy centers between him and the woman who had left him some twelve years before.

My client had had numerous love relationships since then, but none had come to anything because his heart was still closed. Like many people, his heart had been broken and energetically he had simply shut it down. I helped him cut the cords between him and his ex-wife, and used energy healing to reopen his heart. Eventually, his back pain went away and he was able to fall in love again.

If your heart is closed, you are either punishing yourself or protecting yourself. You could be punishing yourself for something that happened so long ago that you yourself may have even forgotten. As a kinesiologist, I like to identify if a person's heart is open or closed. If your heart is closed, I like to find out if you are punishing yourself or protecting yourself, and why. You could be punishing yourself for a childhood event. It could be something that happened even recently.

If this is the case, you may have a subconscious belief that you are a bad person or that you don't deserve to be loved, either unconditionally or even at all. If you look at things from the God view, this is not the case. Of course you deserve to be loved. Of course your soul is innocent and good—no matter what you have done, what you have said, where you have been, or whatever troubles you have gotten embroiled in. You are a child of God and, therefore, deserve to allow the light of God's love to come streaming into your heart.

If you are protecting yourself, maybe you have been hurt at some point, perhaps very badly. Some of the most coldhearted people you will meet are just protecting themselves. Deep down, they are not really coldhearted; they are just afraid. The thing to do is just to realize that if God is all there is, it's all God and, therefore, it's all good.

Even the times in your life when you have been deeply hurt, incredibly abused, robbed, or taken advantage of, there was some divine reason for it. You may be smart enough to figure out what that reason is at the time, it may take you years to develop that perspective, or you may never figure it out at all. However, the reason is always there.

If you are the type of person who defends himself or herself, then you are protecting yourself from being attacked. But no love of God can ever attack you. At the end of the day, it is actually safer to stop defending yourself against life. The love of God shines equally upon all of us, even those of us who think He/She/It has forgotten us. This is a mistake purely of understanding and misperception. At the end of the day, there is nothing but love, as there is nothing but God.

So back to you trying to protect yourself. Don't do it, I say! Allow yourself to have a completely undefended experience of life, and allow the light of God to flow through your life freely, openly, and with renewed purpose. This is the essence of unconditional love.

CHAPTER 9. THE SEVEN LAYERS OF THE HEART

"What do you find in the average middle-aged man of woman? You're likely to see disharmony and unequal spin rates in the chakras. The slower ones would be causing parts of the body to deteriorate, while the faster ones would be causing nervousness, anxiety, and exhaustion. In short, chakras spinning either too quickly or too slowly produce ill health. From this we gather that the Five Rites coordinate, even enhance, the spinning of the seven energy centers of the human body; they help distribute pure life force energy to the endocrine glands and in turn to the body's organs and processes. When this happens, the result is longevity and rejuvenation."

—PETER KELDER

I remember years ago stumbling upon the set of exercises known as the Tibetan Rites. You can read about them in a book called *Ancient Secrets of the Fountain of Youth* by Peter Kelder (Harbor Press, 1985), or visit my website, *www.totalfitness.net*, to see pictures and videos.

I was at a conference studying acupressure when this group of lovely ladies found out that I was teaching yoga. They showed me the Tibetan Rites and told me how much they loved practicing them. I just started doing the five exercises because the lovely ladies told me how much energy they got from doing them. I had no idea just how much the exercises would change my life.

For one, as I began practicing the exercise that looks like a dynamic moving yoga camel pose, I began to notice a pain in my chest. At first, I thought that I had pulled a muscle. I remember poking around at the muscles in my chest area before I realized that the pain I had been feeling was actually energetic. My heart had never been that open. Simply practicing the Tibetan Rites had opened my heart.

I had loved many people and pets by that time, I loved what I did and where I was in my life at the time but, energetically, all seven layers of my heart chakra had never been that open.

Let me step back a minute to talk about chakras. For those of you who may not be familiar, these are vortexes of energy that correspond to your endocrine glands. Energy healers can use a pendulum to tell whether your chakras are either open or closed. If your chakras are open and spinning clockwise, you are able to absorb energy from your environment, feel vital and alive, and your endocrine glands are healthy. If your chakras are closed or spinning counterclockwise, you may have trouble with low energy and have under-functioning endocrine glands.

Although much has been written about the chakras by many other authors, I would like to provide my perspective from teaching about these energy centers and also healing them for many years.

First, it is very helpful to understand the way that energy flows through your body. Energy enters your body through the crown of your head. There is a vertical electrical current, your hara line, that runs from above the crown of your head through your physical body down into the center of the Earth.

Your hara line feeds energy into vortexes called chakras. There are seven major chakras, and depending on who you listen to, countless others. I have studied with other healers who believe you have as many as twenty-seven chakras extending well above your head, connecting you into the cosmos.

The chakras feed energy into your acupuncture meridians. Your acupuncture meridians feed energy into your organs. And, finally, your organs feed energy into your muscles.

So, if you have a health problem or you are not feeling as happy as you could be, the question becomes where along this complex system your energy may not be flowing as efficiently as it could. Physical illness may shut down your chakras, but so may any emotional, mental, or spiritual issue. If your chakras are not functioning properly, they may literally be clogged with old energy and information that you have subconsciously held on to.

As an energy healer, I am able to clean out this old energy and rebuild your chakra. These energy centers may be spinning counterclockwise, as opposed to clockwise, which is what happens when we are mentally, emotionally, and physically healthy.

On the other hand, when your hara line is open, you are connected to the Earth and to the divine at the same time, your chakras are all open and balanced, you will feel both grounded and divinely guided, healthy and happy, all in an effortless way.

I believe that keeping your energy system open and healthy is essential for receiving intuitive information, because each chakra allows us to process energy and information of high value.

In the appendix section, you can see a full list of the seven major chakras and their attributes.

Although alternative healers focus primarily on seven chakras corresponding to the seven major endocrine glands, as many as twenty-seven chakras have been discovered.

As I mentioned earlier, there are seven layers of the heart chakra. What are they? The first layer of your heart energy is called the *etheric*. It extends just a few inches beyond your physical body. It's the lowest level of your energy field.

Farther out, the second layer of heart energy is the *emotional heart*. The emotions of the heart are quite complex. When we know who we are, are able to love unconditionally, and laugh a lot, this layer is open and balanced. Forgiveness, compassion, self-esteem, and self-worth are all virtues that strengthen the emotional layer of the heart.

The third layer is the *mental* layer of our heart. This has to do with thoughts and beliefs we have built up about who we are, what life is about, and how we think about our relationships with other people.

The fourth layer is the *astral* level. You can think of this as the higher level of your emotional layer of your heart. It connects you to your spirituality.

The fifth layer is your *etheric template*. I like to think of this as functioning like a cookie cutter or metaprogram—it is the inner design of the heart.

The sixth layer is the *celestial body*. When we connect to this aspect of our hearts, we can experience deep levels of bliss.

The seventh layer is the *causal body*. This layer contains all the other layers. It contains our true soul.

Keeping the energy centers we call chakras open and balanced is absolutely essential to being intuitive and also being healthy and fully alive. Why is this? The chakras are not only vortexes of energy, they are also centers for psychic reception. They are places where we receive information and, if they are closed, we will not be able to access the full power of our intuitive gifts.

The Tibetan Rites is a simple series of five yoga exercises anyone can do that will open all the chakras. I know because I have tested the chakras of countless clients both before and after performing the Tibetan Rites, and I have found these exercises to be highly effective.

In addition to the Tibetan Rites, you could also follow a daily practice of either yoga, tai chi, or qi gong, as these exercises also open and balance the energy system of the body. After practicing the Tibetan Rites for a few weeks, the pain in my chest that was not related to any muscle soreness went away.

I did not know at the time what energetic block I had been releasing. Like many other people, there were plenty of ways my heart had been hurt. Often we hold so much grief and pain in our energy bodies, we can't even recall what it was all about. The beauty of performing these exercises is that they allow the blocks to be released in a nonverbal but complete way. Finally free, we can be in the present moment and feel more at peace.

Chapter 10. How Do You Know If Your Heart Is Open?

"Trust your intuition and be guided by love."

—Charles Eisenstein

I remember one time years ago working with a client in my office. I had him hooked up to an EKG device, a simple monitor on my computer that showed his electrocardiogram, or electric activity of his heart, and taught him how he could change it with his thoughts and feelings. I was working with him to lower his blood pressure, and I was trying to help him with the physical aspects of his heart. I asked him to think of someone he actually loved. He confessed he couldn't think of anyone. "Think of a pet, then," I suggested. Still, no luck. Finally, he admitted he loved his sailboat. That was the crack in him where the light could finally get in.

Although my client had been quite successful

financially, he had been unable to form a long-term, loving relationship. He had recently been married, but his marriage only lasted about a week. The fact that everything fell apart so quickly was a surprise to everyone concerned. He came to me afterward, ostensibly for help with his blood pressure, but he and I both knew that the issues with his heart were more complicated than just his systolic and diastolic pressure.

I remember feeling completely surprised that the only thing he could think of that he really loved was his sailboat.

A graduate of an Ivy League college, he had developed his mind but not the higher intelligence of his heart. You have to feel safe to open your heart, you have to feel safe to feel your feelings, and you have to feel really, really safe in order to share your feelings with another person.

How do you know if your heart is open? You know if you are able to give and receive love. It's that simple. Many people are very loving toward others but don't know how to let love in.

There are many varieties of dysfunction that can lead to a closing of the heart but, if you can think of even one person you actually love and one person whom you allow to love you, there is a crack wide enough to allow the light in.

Everyone has a crack where the light and love can get in. For some of us, this crack may be as wide as a river or as vast as an ocean. For others, it may just be just that: a crack, or a break in the hardened shell of who we have become. But it's there.

How do you know if you have a crack? If there is something that just allows you to recognize that you are broken. That doesn't mean that there is something wrong with you; instead, it means that you are not perfect and that only love can mend you. This would be the love of God, another person, a pet, or the love you experience standing in a beautiful garden. It could be your ability to laugh with your friends at a midnight poker game, or your joy in dancing. It could even be that you feel a little better when you look out your window and see the sun coming up over the horizon.

The crack in you is so deep, maybe even so hidden or complicated, that even you don't quite understand it. Maybe you have even done years of therapy and yet you are aware, your crack is still there. It is love that you need to fill that crack.

Forget being perfect. Just forget about it. Allow that crack to bring in the light of God. As mentioned earlier, there are seven layers to your heart chakra. Maybe you can even find more, but I do believe that there are depths to which you can open your heart; when your heart is fully open you can be the place that love flows through. Even if you think your heart is already open, perhaps there is another small degree to which you can open yourself that might totally revolutionize your experience of life.

This may be your divine purpose, to allow enough love to flow through that your work can come from love, your home can be a place of love, and everyone and everything around you can feel it. We can maintain a healthy, open heart simply by realizing that the energy of one truly loving thought is more powerful than any one thought or feeling of apathy, grief, fear, craving, anger, or pride, and more powerful than all negative feelings combined.

Beginning wherever we are in life, at whatever emotional place we find ourselves in, we can focus on allowing ourselves to feel love wherever we find it. This could be the love for our mother, father, brother, sister, or other family members. It could be love for our friends. It could be love for our pets. It could be love for our partner, our love for all of humanity, the love we express by doing work we enjoy or spending time in a beautiful garden.

If we can only begin with one truly loving thought, that is the place to begin. That one loving feeling will begin to shift our vibration completely.

Chapter 11. How Much Love Is in It?

"Amazing grace! How sweet the sound
That saved a wretch like me!
I once was lost, but now am found:
Was blind, but now I see."

—John Newton

When I begin to evaluate something, one of the questions I ask myself is, "How much love is in it?"

In the *Ion,* Plato argued that there is an unbroken chain between the Divine, the inspiration received by an artist of any kind, and the audience who receives that message.

"In like manner the Muse first of all inspires men herself; and from these inspired persons a chain of other persons is suspended, who take the inspiration," Plato wrote.

It feels to me that the more direct our connection to our deepest core sense of love, whether we are creating anything or witnessing the creation of another, the greater the impact any work of art, no matter how humble it is.

Personally, I can't hear even the first verse of "Amazing Grace" without being moved to tears. I can be in the greatest mood but, upon hearing even the first four lines, tears will start streaming down my face.

This song has always had an effect on me, even as a child, decades before I learned the story about the author John Newton. Understanding his story and the background he went through—pressed into service for the Royal Navy, himself captured as a slave in Africa, then spending years as a slave trader and investor in the same business before becoming an Anglican priest—only deepens the impact of the song for me.

If I am to follow Plato's model, it would appear that Newton was inspired to write "Amazing Grace" from his experiences. But is also clear that his ability to capture the essence of the Divine comes through every time I hear the song. It captivates me and moves me to tears.

I believe that my gardener, Gabe, is inspired because it shows in his work. I always marvel at how both of us can plant violas and get such different results. We each dig a hole in the ground. We both throw in fertilizer. Some years, as a scientific experiment, I planted violas in one area while Gabe planted the same flowers from the same wholesaler in another bed. Gabe's flowers always fared better than mine.

We both love my garden. And, being that this is

my house, you would think I would love my garden even more than Gabe does. But somehow his flowers always grow a little more lushly than the ones I put into the ground. Why is that? I believe it is because of how much love Gabe puts into his work.

Gabe knows exactly where the sun shines and the shade lands on my front lawn. Even though I have lived here for years, he has taught me more about the patterns of the land than I realized before he pointed them out to me. He knows where the soil needs to be enriched, and where I make it a little too rich. He knows when to cut the trees and shrubs back, even though I would be happy to let them grow tall. He knows because he sees how the whole garden works together. He knows that if you let something grow too tall, it might block out the sun on the flowers and how opening the corridor by the side of the house might allow everyone to appreciate the arbor there that much more. Gabe puts so much love into his work that it's obvious.

This is a mark of excellence, of course, but it's not just the excellence that comes from the intellect alone. It's the true knowing that can only come from the heart.

Here is another example from recent memory. My spiritual guidance told me one day that I had to go to my local ACE Hardware on a particular morning. I love the ACE Hardware near my house because the people there are so friendly, whether it's the guy who carefully loads the bags of cypress mulch into my car or the lady behind the cash register who always waits patiently as I fumble to find the ACE Rewards card in my wallet.

When I arrived at ACE that spring morning, I discovered there were only two huge pots of apple blossom double begonias, my absolute favorites; I learned that was going to be all they would have available for the whole year.

I love my garden so much that I knew exactly the right time to show up to get what I needed to put around the fountain by my studio.

But I was distraught to find there didn't seem to be enough double begonias to fill my flower bed. So the lady in the plant department brought me over to the pots of euphorbia, a sparkly white flower with delicate leaves, whose overall effect sounds exactly like it sounds.

Being as there weren't enough begonias, I bought the euphorbia to go with them. I came home, carefully broke apart the two plastic pots and, bit by bit, gingerly pulled apart those two plants into sixteen divisions. Within a very short period of time, you could hardly tell that I had parted two plants because the entire flower bed exploded into something even more magical than I had originally intended: pink double blossoms with a wisp of shimmering white euphorbia, like a halo around my fountain.

There may be some other clues as to why Gabe's plants do so well. In his books, *Messages from Water* and *The Hidden Messages in Water*, author Masaru Emoto describes how water molecules respond to their environment. Simply writing the word "love" on a bottle of water changes its molecular structure. Plants are 90 percent water, and I believe that they react immediately to the energy surrounding them.

During a period of intense stress in my life, I was dismayed to see how every one of the orchids in my studio became afflicted with mealy bugs. Many of my cultivars had bloomed continuously for as long as five years, and suddenly they were all covered. Next to scale insects, mealy bugs are probably the most difficult to control pests afflicting orchids, weakening the leaves, buds and flowers and covering everything with a dew that attracts ants and mold.

I understood immediately the connection between my own emotional state and the sudden downfall of my orchids. Deeply troubled, I wrote to Don Dennis, the orchid grower in Scotland, for help.

"Mealy bugs are like the difference between someone saying bad things about you and someone throwing flames at you," Don wrote me back.

Trying as I might, I was unable to eliminate the mealy bugs completely until I disposed of all my orchids and completely renovated my entire studio. In fact, it was the distress of my orchids that convinced me of the absolute necessity of clearing out all the old energy by giving away two-thirds of my books and belongings, painting from floor to ceiling, and installing new carpet. I love my orchids so much I was determined to recreate a happy environment for them.

We humans and other animals are about 75 percent water. In the same manner, I believe our living tissue comes into immediate harmony when placed in an environment of love and care.

On my fiftieth birthday, my friend Lee Townsend

made me a cake. It was so good that everyone at the party asked for two and even three pieces. Even though I don't usually eat seconds on cake, I asked for another piece and was sorely disappointed when my plate was removed before I could finish it!

Lee had invented a recipe for organic, gluten-free coconut cake. It had taken her a total of two days to make the cake, including visiting the grocer to buy the actual coconuts, taking a hammer to break them apart, and using a fork and various other lethal-looking instruments to extract the meat of the nut.

She kept her recipe a secret. She knew that it was hers and hers alone, not just because she had come up with the proportions but because all of her years as a mother, organic chef, and healthy eater had gone into her intention of making the best cake possible. That cake had so much love in it that you could taste it.

You may not know the story behind why a song or a garden is so beautiful or why a cake tastes so good but, if you pay enough attention, you can tell how much love is in it.

Although you may not be able to quantify just what it is exactly, you will be able to feel the difference, because the divine energy that inspired the artist that created it will flow through to you, the receiver, in a way that touches your heart.

CHAPTER 12. SEARCHING FOR LOVE

"Spiritual evolution occurs as the result of removing obstacles and not actually acquiring anything new."

—DAVID HAWKINS, M.D.

Like most women, despite all the love I received from my grandmother and my professor from college, I spent many years looking for love, as if it were something to be discovered. I dated all the wrong guys. I looked in all the wrong places. I even married the wrong person once, as I mentioned before, and then married the right guy until it wasn't right anymore. Like most people, I thought that love was something outside of myself. I thought it was something you had to go looking for.

My early attempts at searching for love landed me in not one but many wrong and painful places. I spent two years at a YWCA support group for battered women in Nashville, Tennessee. Every meeting, women from the projects, from the fancy houses with maids and lots of silver, me, and everybody else in between, sat there and went over the "Wheel of Power and Control." This was a diagram explaining all the various ways, including physical violence, that women who thought they were in a loving relationship would in fact be controlled and were not in a loving relationship.

Every week, the facilitators would draw a large circle on a big piece of paper and all of us would have to try to remember how to fill it in. Given that I sat there week after week, month after month, for two years, you would think I would have it all memorized by now. However, when you are in an abusive situation it is a difficult thing to face.

As a dear friend of mine said to me in recent years: "Fool me once, shame on me. Fool me 100 times, it's so painful, I can't even bear looking at it."

Intimidation; emotional abuse; male privilege; using money; using the children; minimizing, blaming, and denying; isolation; coercion and threats; sexual abuse; and physical abuse: it all felt so uncomfortable but, at the same time, so familiar. During the time I was attending the support group, about the best thing I read on the subject basically said this: when a child grows up in an abusive household, it is easier for the child to come to the conclusion that there is something wrong with him or her than it is to face the fact that mommy or daddy actually doesn't love him or her.

And I had indeed come to the conclusion that I was damaged goods and that nobody would ever love the real me. I didn't think I deserved to be loved.

I had bought into the idea that there were, indeed, many things wrong with me.

However, I am a can-do type of person. I have the belief that I can fix anything, given the time, money, and resources. I had a bad first marriage, but I thought at first I could fix it. I got my husband to go to the support group for men who hit people. I went to the support group for women. After less than two years, I realized that I was either going to kill him, kill myself, or get out of the marriage. I wisely chose the latter.

I had to face the fact that, in reality, I am not able to fix, heal, or control a lot of things in my life. As I was facing up to his painful picture in my marriage, I began to realize what had actually happened to me growing up.

Growing up the daughter of a successful ophthalmologist in Savannah, Georgia, it appeared to the outside world that I had everything I could ever want or need. However, I remember my father beating me and kicking me on the floor until I urinated on myself while my mother was watching.

As I began healing myself, I visited a chiropractor who took an X-ray of my head. Even though I am not a chiropractor and not an expert at X-rays, I saw very clearly a break in my skull on the right side extending toward my nose.

"You have asthma, don't you?" the chiropractor asked me, explaining that the head injury would have resulted in me having great difficulty with breathing. I had spent years with various kinds of inhalers and taking shots for all my allergies. Looking starkly at the X-ray of my head sent me back to a traditional therapist to talk in detail about what had actually happened to me while growing up. It wasn't a fun discussion.

After those two years at the YWCA support group, I had admitted defeat. What really got me was the time I spent volunteering to babysit for the little children of the other women in the support group. I would go to the group home at the battered women's shelter and babysit while the other women went to their support group meetings.

Even though their children would often be one or two years old, I could tell they had been very badly affected by growing up in an abusive household. Even though they were mere babies, they bore all the signs of abuse themselves.

I realized that it would not be safe for me to bring a child into an abusive marriage, and that if it wasn't safe for a child, it was not right for me either. So I pulled up my socks and moved out.

During this time, I made a list of all the horrible things that had happened to me.

It was so long it was absolutely ridiculous, I thought. I determined right then and there that I wanted my life to be better. I wanted to experience actual love and happiness.

I had no idea how I was going to go about doing that, but I made up my mind that I wanted to experience something better. I quit my regular job and started doing what I thought I wanted to do when I was growing up—write plays—and I fell in love with my second husband. Things began to feel better.

Then one day I remember a friend of mine telling me, "Catherine, you would love yoga." Cheeky as I was, I replied, "Yoga is for wimps," something I would obviously never say today. I began practicing yoga with a videotape in my living room. I didn't have a yoga mat and kept slipping around on my carpet. The people in the video seemed to be able to keep their feet steady in the poses. I wasn't accustomed to spending much money on myself, so it was a huge deal when I finally bought a yoga mat to keep my feet from slipping on the carpet.

All of a sudden, after practicing yoga with a video for a month in my living room, my spiritual beliefs radically changed. The church I had been attending every week didn't feel right anymore. I wasn't sure how that happened, as nothing in the videotape included any discussion about God or even spirituality. The only hint was that the instructor encouraged me to breathe deeply and lie down for five minutes at the end of my practice—something I found very challenging at the time, as my mind would race and I didn't know how to find the silence inside.

I didn't know what I was doing, but I knew I had stumbled upon something that I loved to do. Like the people we love so much in our lives who show up unexpectedly just when we need them, yoga showed up on a thirteen-dollar videotape and completely changed my life.

I thought I had been searching for a person, or a way of feeling. What I received at that time from the practice of yoga was a tool to open myself on all levels so that the love of God for all that is could flow through me.

Although there are endless benefits to practicing yoga, I believe that at its root what the practice of yoga did for me was open up all my energy channels so that I could finally feel deeply connected to—as opposed to alone, apart, and separate from—all that is.

When we feel alone, apart, and separate, we look around at other people and feel threatened, unsure, or insecure. When we finally feel this deep sense of connection, our fears begin to dissipate.

Since beginning my practice of yoga, I have found many other ways to open my energy channels. I believe that qi gong and tai chi are equally helpful in this regard. So is receiving Reiki, a form of hands-on energy healing which balances the energy system.

As we open our energy channels, we can cease the process of searching for love and begin the process of becoming an actual channel for love, allowing the force that drives the growth of flowers, summer rain, autumn wind, and winter snow to flow through us at the cellular level.

Chapter 13. There Are Many Ways To Open Your Heart

"When we speak of God, we speak of one and all, for all, in all, through all and of all."

—Baird T. Spalding

There are many ways to open your heart. As I mentioned in the last chapter, I have found yoga, tai chi, and qi gong as great ways to open my heart. You may have other activities that you may involve yourself in, but just be sure that these exercises give you the desired result: greater flow from the heart.

It is important to open your heart if you really want to be intuitive, so let's take some time to talk about how to do this. The first step is to recognize if you are protecting yourself or punishing yourself. If your heart is closed, chances are you either protecting yourself or punishing yourself. Perhaps you are even doing both.

If you are protecting yourself, other people may feel a wall around you. That wall will be invisible, for sure, but it will still be there. You will have trouble letting anyone in to know the true you. You may feel that wall yourself and other people will also. They may even feel like they bounce off of it if they try to get too close to you.

If you are protecting yourself, you may have a subconscious belief that if you let anyone in, they might not like you or end up judging you harshly. You will notice a lack of close friendships or intimate companions in your life.

On the road to leading a more heart-centered life, affirmations have always been helpful. By simply stating our intention to be more productive, to generate more love, or even to establish close, intimate ties with another person, we begin the process of transforming our relationship to ourselves.

Here is an example of an affirmation I might use if I wanted to release a wall of protection:

TO KNOW MYSELF IS TO LOVE MYSELF.

IT IS SAFE TO BE WHO I TRULY AM ON ALL
LEVELS NOW.

GOD LOVES ME.

I AM LOVABLE.

I AM OPEN TO GIVING AND RECEIVING LOVE ON ALL LEVELS.

If you place your hand over your heart as you repeat these affirmations, you can actually feel the power in these words. This opening of your heart begins the process of tapping into your highest intelligence and intuition.

The second possibility if your heart is closed is that you could be punishing yourself. People punish themselves all the time. You could be overworking yourself, spending too much time exercising, overeating, in the throes of an addiction to alcohol or drugs, or practicing any number of self-defeating behaviors. You could notice if you are punishing yourself by paying attention to your self-talk. For example, "How stupid/small/insignificant/unlovable/wrong/damaged/no good I am," you may be telling yourself. If you are punishing yourself, find a way to forgive yourself.

Many people don't understand what forgiveness truly is. When you forgive someone, that doesn't mean you now like or even approve of what he or she has done. When you forgive someone, you are willing to let go of resentment, bitterness, hatred, or revenge. You realize how poisonous these emotions are on all levels.

When you forgive someone, you let him or her off the hook. You realize that we are all doing the best we can at the time. And, at the end of the day, you realize that there are no mistakes. That's right: even mistakes aren't really mistakes! It's all good. Ultimately, it's all for your benefit, if you view your entire life like a personalized self-study course in spiritual development. You are engaging in learning the lesson right now, right in this moment, learning exactly whatever it is you are here to learn. For some people, forgiving other people may be easier than forgiving themselves. You can start forgiving yourself with this simple statement:

I LOVE MYSELF.

I KNOW GOD LOVES ME.

I ALLOW THE LIGHT AND LOVE OF GOD
TO FLOW THROUGH ME, TO LIFT ME UP
AND TO FILL MY MIND, BODY, AND SPIRIT.

I AM FREE.

The most important person ever to forgive is yourself. That is because whatever we really think, feel, or believe about ourselves gets projected out onto the world and other people. Once you forgive yourself, then it will be much easier to forgive other people. You will be able to let other people off the hook, and other people can be free around you.

I will tell you a funny story about how I really learned the true meaning of forgiveness. I was teaching yoga one evening. It had been a terrible day—one of those days when you wish you never had gotten out of bed. The person doing my accounting, had misplaced a client's check. The client was very upset with me and called and yelled at me for an hour, even though it was not my mistake. I took it all in and apologized.

That same day, a credit card that had been lost was later discovered to have been stolen. The person who stole the credit card racked up thousands of dollars in bills that had to be sorted out. As the hours wore on, the stress kept piling up. Then, at the end of the day, I thought, *Thank God; now I get to go teach yoga.* I showed up at the room at the church where I usually teach yoga, only to discover that a women's group had gotten mixed up and taken over our room.

We being yogis, we graciously agreed to move to another room. After about fifteen minutes, and after hauling our mats to the new location, we all had settled down and were practicing our poses. A representative of the women's group came to me, apologized profusely, and let me know they had created the space in the room so we could practice our yoga. We all trooped back to our spot.

At last, I thought, *all is well in the world.* Finally, as usual, I guided everyone into meditation. Also as usual, I shut my eyes and meditated along with my students. For just a brief moment, I felt calm and at peace again. When I opened my eyes, however, I felt something amiss.

Outside in the hallway, I saw a priest from the church. He was practically foaming at the mouth. Apparently, during meditation, one of my yoga students had gotten up from his mat, gone into the hallway, and started a fight with a member of the women's group, calling her "a fat cow." Now, I believe probably the worst thing you could ever call a woman is a fat cow!

Horrified, I apologized profusely to the priest. I also apologized to the woman, who was acutely embarrassed. I could not believe that any student of mine could have practiced yoga and gotten up out of meditation to insult someone.

The next day, the story only intensified. The staff at the church wanted me to eject the member from my yoga class. It turned out that individual was also a member of the church, so the situation only became more complicated. I knew that person really needed to practice yoga to overcome stress.

Finally, I had a phone conversation with the assistant to the head of the church. "Fortunately," I said to her, "sainthood is not required for membership in yoga class. We are all just trying to calm down and be better people." She got it immediately.

The individual who had caused the ruckus apologized to me personally but, even before then, that gesture had become unnecessary, as I had already forgiven him. A few days later, I was playing with my angel cards and I drew the Angel of Forgiveness. I realized that I had been blessed with this very peculiar little drama so that the Angel of Forgiveness could visit me and teach me in a way that I would never forget.

When we see other people through the eyes of love, everything looks upside down. Everything that seems awful on this immediate earthly plane often looks quite the opposite on the spiritual level.

I remember once being at a very large convention. There were several thousand people in the audience. I was sitting next to a woman, who turned to me and said, "I have no idea who you are or what you do, but I know you are supposed to help me." It turned out that the lady was a professional therapist.

In addition to that, she was an adopted child. All she knew about her biological parents was that her birth mother was a "loser," a drug addict who had given birth out of wedlock and had given up her child shortly after giving birth.

When we looked at the situation from another perspective, it turned out that the birth mother had a soul contract to give birth to my client. One of the aspects of my spiritual training became clear early on: oftentimes, when a soul wants to be incarnated, there may be many attempts before an actual birth is successful. Many fetuses are spontaneously aborted through no fault of the mother. So many souls that are trying to be born have to find another ride.

My client, the therapist, had a big reason for getting here. So she had taken the only ride she could get. The birth mother had literally agreed to give up her life so that the daughter could be born. Giving up her daughter had been so painful for her that the birth mother never recovered.

So, in the end, rather than being a "loser," on the soul level, the birth mother was actually an unselfish giver. The therapist was so thankful to have obtained this new perspective about her mother; this gave her new ideas about how important her life actually is.

In another case, I had a client who had been

physically abused as a child. Her father was a very angry alcoholic. My client had stood up to him, and often stood between him and her younger siblings. She literally took the beating in their place.

When we looked at the situation from the soul level, her father had agreed to teach my client how to be a strong, independent person. And that she was.

Take all mistakes for love, because there actually are no mistakes.

CHAPTER 14. HEART OPENERS

"In resonance all fluid systems are united. I say that no matter where in the galaxy they may be, all fluid systems function as basically one body or organ of intelligence."

—EMILIE CONRAD

I am quite serious about keeping my energy open and balanced because I understand how important it is to be open to God and grounded to the Earth at the same time. When we are connected to the God Source and the Earth simultaneously, we maintain our vertical energy connection to the boundless supply of consciousness and information.

If you are grounded but not connected to the divine, you can't get spiritual, psychic, and intuitive information. People who have a good earth connection but are shut off from their divinity may do a great job navigating the practical aspects of life, but their souls may long for something deeper.

If you are connected to the divine but ungrounded, watch out: you can get yourself into lots of trouble, not just with misunderstanding where you are in the earthly plane, but in becoming psychically overloaded. People who are connected to the divine but lack a good earth connection may live their life a short distance from their body. They may appear a bit spacey, even if they are otherwise brilliant. They could have trouble with whole body coordination. Without a good mind-body connection, they may not be able to tell when they are full wihle eating, when they hurt or are feeling sick ,or when they need to stop what they are doing to take a rest.

This was my case for many years. I was terribly ungrounded. My energy was so pulled up out of my body that when I first started studying how to use intuition for healing, my teachers advised me, "Don't go up, only go down." By "pulled up" I mean that I wasn't actually at home in my body. I never needed to learn how to connect to the divine; that was something I had down pat. What I needed was to connect to my body in a practical way.

A healer who did regular energy work with me said, "When I started working with you, I couldn't actually find you!" When a person is accustomed to being abused, it can feel safer for the soul to leave the body and view the situation from a distance. However, being ungrounded and out of body is not an ideal situation.

When you are out of body, lacking a good mind-body connection, you may experience the following symptoms:

- Inability to know when you are tired, hungry, full, or in need of help
- Physically uncoordinated
- Disconnected from your true feelings
- Out of touch with the feelings of others, since you have to be in touch with yourself before you can actually be in touch with others
- Racing around with little awareness
- Adrenal burnout
- Anxious
- Easily thrown off balance
- Spacey
- May develop multiple physical illnesses and not even know you are unwell

I had been exercising for many years to try to connect back into my body, even though when I started I could exercise as much as three hours a day and not realize why I was so tired. Through years of practice, I have pulled myself back into my body. Although I have discovered that I need near-daily movement to maintain my mind-body connection, I can exercise moderately for an hour or less and maintain a good connection to the here and now.

During that time of my life I was in my mid-thirties, and I knew intuitively that I was struggling to connect into my body and feel safe in the here and the now.

I understood that I was suffering from a serious eating disorder—the second one of my lifetime, as I had also been anorexic at age sixteen.

As a teenager, I had gotten down to around ninety pounds. My parents solved that problem by telling me how ugly I was. So I began to eat again, this time ballooning up to 150 pounds.

I had fortunately achieved a normal weight most of my life, but after getting out of the support group for battered women and leaving an abusive marriage, I found myself bingeing when I reached my thirties. I would go into a Shoney's restaurant, look at the breakfast bar and think, *that's just not enough food!*

Even though I did not want to overeat, I would be someplace and suddenly and unexpectedly experience a piercing panic attack of no known origin. Often it felt like 1,000 volts of electricity running through an ordinary light socket, as if I had been struck by lightning. Eating would help calm and ground me. Often, after such an episode of panic followed by overeating, I would then fall asleep suddenly.

It was difficult to describe these episodes to so-called "normal" people, who didn't seem to have trouble handling the energy of being alive. I realized that I was sensitive to just about everything in the modern world—cell phones, computers, virtually any kind of EMF device, body scanners at the airport, fluorescent lights, strange smells. If I was driving a car, I could feel the cars driving down the expressway next to me.

It wasn't just electrical or modern gadget phenomena that affected me. While walking in my neighborhood during a drought, I could literally feel the trees and shrubs dying from lack of water. One summer when the drought in Atlanta was particularly bad, I felt awful for months as I could feel the effects on the plant life so extremely. Even if I sat in my house and meditated, I could feel the vibration of the cars driving down the road next to my house.

In addition to food, another way I would self-medicate was through exercise. I knew very well that working out for more than one hour was not ideal, but if I was moving my body, I knew I would feel calmer both during the exercise and afterward. It almost didn't matter what I was doing—running, walking, lifting weights, practicing yoga—so long as I was in constant motion. Then I could tolerate the experience of being alive.

I was either stuffing my feelings or running away from them, even if I didn't understand at the time exactly what those feelings actually were. Of course, the side effects of these behaviors wrought havoc on my physical health. I developed chronic fatigue syndrome and a whole host of other problems so extensive I don't even want to remember.

At the end of the day, I have had to learn how to become strong enough to handle my extreme sensitivity. As an extremely sensitive person, you may be processing literally 400 to 600 times more energy and information than someone without extrasensory gifts. This may take a toll on your nervous system. When you are an extremely sensitive person, you either become grounded—centered and strong, mentally, emotionally, spiritually, and physically—or you find yourself unable to function in everyday life.

I like to explain it this way when I am speaking to other highly sensitive people: "If you own a Ferrari, you better learn how to drive it; otherwise, you can get in trouble in a hurry." Even though I have become strong and healthy, I prefer a quiet life, working out of my home, rooting myself in my garden, with my orchids and in my studio, doing all I can to keep my stress level low.

I also do practical, mundane things like clean my own house. There is nothing like getting down on your hands and knees and scrubbing your floor to make you feel grounded! The hours I spend mopping, dusting, vacuuming, polishing, and cleaning bring me more into the peace of the moment than I could have previously imagined.

In his book, *Care of the Soul: Guide for Cultivating Depth and Sacredness in Everyday Life* (Piatkus, 2012), author Thomas Moore writes, "To the soul, the most minute details and the most ordinary activities, carried out with mindfulness and art, have an effect far beyond their apparent insignificance."

Once you have learned to let down the walls around you, forgive yourself, and you have begun the endless practice of forgiving others (since we are all human, we all tend to get our feelings hurt from time to time, or get angry or disappointed, so forgiveness is a constant practice), you can probably feel more love already flowing through your heart.

If you are like many others, you may have been searching for love outside of yourself for many years, thinking that it is something to be acquired, just like something you might get a good deal on at the thrift store if you are lucky.

Energy exercises like yoga, tai chi, and qi gong can

go a long way to open your heart, even if you don't do the deeper work of forgiveness. Why is that? Yoga, tai chi, and qi gong are energy practices designed to open and balance the energy channels in your body. If you are going to be intuitive, you have to maintain a very balanced energy system, and it has to be open and stay appropriately open for you to receive information without blowing your circuits. Find an activity that will help you balance your energy system, and you will start to feel the intuitive gifts start filtering through—and you'll probably cultivate more love in the process!

In Chinese medicine, the heart is the emperor of the body. When the heart is open and balanced, that is a pretty good indication that a person is healthy and radiant. In yoga theory, the heart is believed to be the connection point between the physical body and the spiritual body.

Your arms are an extension of your heart, so everything that you do with your hands comes out of your heart, whether it be making a meal for others, beading or knitting (like I do), writing a letter to a friend, or hugging a loved one. Tai chi and qi gong are based on the Chinese medical practice of acupuncture. Both tai chi and qi gong balance the acupuncture system, so if you practice these arts, you know that not only will you be getting a good cardiovascular workout through deep breathing, you will also be balancing the acupuncture meridian for your heart.

In yoga, my favorite heart-opening exercises are backbends: wheel, cobra, camel, locust pose, up dog, and sage twist all fit the bill. Any deep breathing exercise will also balance your heart because of the intimate connection between your lungs and your heart. I like to practice heart-opening exercises every time I practice yoga because they feel so good.

Scientific research shows that your heart activity governs your brain activity. An EKG, or electrocardiogram, measures the rate and regularity of your heartbeats. An EEG, or electroencephalogram, measures voltage fluctuations in the neurons of your brain. It is not commonly known outside of scientific circles that the heart sends more signals to the brain, rather than the other way around.

Your brain continuously responds to your heart. When you are in positive states of love or appreciation, you operate at a higher level of what is called *coherence*. Through coherence your entire body systems synchronize and operate at a higher functioning level. That means your heart waves actually govern your brain waves. In fact, it is said that your EKG is sixty times more powerful than your EEG.

When you practice deep yogic breathing, your EKG and your EEG can come into *entrainment*. That means there is a deep level of synchronization between your heart and your brain. When you are in entrainment, you access your deepest intelligence, which is the kind of knowing that I want to teach you about. Even if you are not physically fit or very flexible, you can find energy exercises that open your heart.

Chapter 15. Laughing

"The most wasted of all days is one without laughter."

—E. E. CUMMINGS

One of my favorite ways to open my heart is by laughing. I don't actually think I am very funny, but I love to go to the comedy club. I like to go with a good friend and laugh my head off at all the stupid jokes. In fact, if I ever get depressed, going to the comedy club is one of my favorite forms of therapy.

I also like to watch comedies when I go to the movie theater or on my movie player at home. My favorite comedian is probably Steve Martin, seconded only by Eddie Murphy. Even if you can't talk yourself into practicing tai chi, yoga, or qi gong, you can probably talk yourself into laughing a lot.

Beware the humorless. People who are all too serious are missing a key aspect of intelligence, which is perspective! At the end of the day, things are not all that serious, even death. Even when a person passes away, they are still actually with you.

I remember being really sick years ago. The doctor I was seeing at the time was worried that I might have a heart problem. When I arrived at the cardiologist's office, everybody looked at me as though I was out of place. I was relatively young. I was thin. I probably seemed to have a good complexion from good blood circulation—I exercised regularly. I was so alarmed that a doctor might think I had heart problems that I too began to get worried.

Sitting in the cardiologist's office, all by myself with my feet dangling off the table, I had a vision of my grandfather, who had passed away years before. In my vision, he was even wearing a shirt I had given him for one of his birthdays. He patted my hand and told me that everything was okay. He was right.

The cardiologist looked puzzled. He had had me hooked up to a device and could not find anything wrong with my heart. He too wondered why anyone would have sent me there.

Later, I thought it was ridiculous that I needed an expensive visit to the cardiologist just to get a message from Spirit! I had a little laugh about it. I just needed to see my grandfather and get the message that I was being totally looked after, and that everything would always be okay.

If you are having trouble thinking of anything to laugh about, there is an energy exercise you can do that will help.

First, sit on the floor. You can put a pillow underneath you if you like to be more comfortable.

Put one hand on your heart, and with your other hand reach out. Imagine that you are looking into the eyes of someone you care about.

Focus on your heart area. Fill your heart with a deep green light—a healing color for the heart. Take a deep breath in. As you exhale, say, "Ha!"

Inhale and change your hands.

Now the other hand is over your heart. The other arm is extending. As you exhale, repeat, "Ha!"

Keep focusing on your heart, inhaling and exhaling with the "Ha!" sound.

Visualize your heart opening up and, as you do, feel the balance between giving and receiving in your life.

Chapter 16. Green and Pink

"The things you have around you are not really yours. They are material manifestations of an infinite abundance."

—Stuart Wilde

There are many techniques in healing that are surprisingly simple but profound. One of them is the use of color. The healing colors for the heart include green and/or pink. Color therapy works on the spiritual body. Although it seems simple, its effects are deep and profound. If you want to heal your heart or open your heart, you can visualize green light or pink light (whatever feels most appropriate to you) pouring forth from your heart.

How do I know that green is actually the healing color for the heart? I remember years ago, when I was studying healing work in Canada, someone brought in a professional to take photographs of our auras. Although many people had an aura that seemed like a cloud, my aura was completely clear. You could see the colors of each chakra. My heart was filled with green light and it was very big.

"Whatever happens in your life from now on," the man who read my aura told me, "you will be okay. Your chakras are all open and balanced. You can handle anything life brings you."

I can only speculate as to why my chakras were so open. However, by that time in my life, I had been practicing yoga and qi gong regularly, often as many as ten or twelve hours a week. It is my experience when evaluating other people who practice energy exercises that these ancient practices keep the energy system of the body open and radiantly healthy.

In addition, by that point, I had done a great deal of personal healing. I had overcome my asthma, eating disorders, chronic fatigue, gotten off lithium and antidepressants, forgiven my father, and become a happier person. When we heal ourselves physically, emotionally, mentally, and spiritually, that information shows up in our energy field quite clearly; there are no further blocks to keeping the chakras open and balanced.

One of the things I do as a professional healer is make jewelry for my clients. Whenever I do, I always tune in to their energy and use colors and gemstones specifically designed to heal each person.

I remember years ago that one of my clients hired me to make a necklace for her mother for a Christmas present. I made a very elaborate piece with pearls and a big clasp. Although my client's mother loved her necklace, she had arthritis and had trouble with the clasp. So I made her another necklace for free.

I waited until she accompanied my client to her session, and then gave her the necklace personally. It was green and full of gemstones of various hues specifically to heal her heart.

"How did you know?" the mother asked me. "I just got out of the hospital from a heart operation!" I had no idea. I just knew, intuitively, when I thought of my client's mother, that she needed green.

Green gemstones that I have used to heal the heart include green aventurine, emerald, green tourmaline, malachite, chrysoprase, jade, amazonite, and chrysocolla.

Pink may be what you need for your heart instead of green. Rose quartz is one of the premier gemstones for healing the heart. Although it is a simple, inexpensive, and readily available gemstone, its effects are quite profound. It is the gemstone I use most often if I am using crystals to heal the heart. Rose-colored tourmaline will also benefit your heart, as will rhodochrosite, rhodonite, and pink sapphire.

My understanding and experience of gemstones is that they work by the quality of resonation. When we use a gemstone in healing work or wear a gemstone, our energies begin to resonate with the specific vibration of the stone we are wearing.

Since every person is a vibrational interference pattern (V.I.P.), gemstones and the specific colors they hold can have a surprisingly strong effect. Rose quartz opens the heart chakra and allows you to feel love for yourself and the entire universe. To me, it embodies the four kinds of healthy love expressed in the Greek words *agape, eros, philia,* and *storge.* It seems to soften the boundaries that keep one from experiencing unconditional love—both giving it out and receiving it.

Many of us think of love as an emotion or feeling. We can certainly feel love. However, it is my experience that when we use subtle remedies such as gemstones, flower essences, alchemy herbs, essential oils, and colored lights, we can open the energy center of the heart and, in this space of deep connection and openness, we can both give and receive love naturally. Love becomes less of something to try to look for and more simply a way of being in the world.

Chapter 17. Carrying Baby Pictures

"Nothing in the world is more common than unsuccessful people with talent, leave the house before you find something worth staying in for."

—Banksy

When you look at a baby human or a baby animal, it is natural to be filled with love.

"How cute! How adorable!" Everything babies do, from the moment they open their eyes, seems like an act of awe and wonder.

You are not really a noun; you are a verb. You are not really a person; you are a soul in action. You are your embryo, you are your baby, you are your child, you are your adult, and you are your spirit when you pass through this body through this lifetime. One of the simplest ways to reconnect with your heart and the love you naturally have for yourself is to look at your own baby pictures.

No matter what mistakes you may have made in

your life up until now, if you looked at your eyes in your baby pictures, you would be able to reconnect with your unblemished character.

As a little girl I had buckteeth from my constant habit of sucking my thumb. I carried around a big blue bunny rabbit. It helped me tremendously when, as an adult, my brother had a little girl named Sarah Jane; everybody said Sarah Jane looked just like I did when I was a young child. From the time she was two, her wispy hair, quirky personality, and her love of art and making things reminded me of who I was at her age.

I remember being on a ferry in Scotland on the way to the Isle of Gigha. I had just met another healer from Finland named Nina Hovik. I felt I had just discovered my soul twin. Nina channels. She practices Reiki. Her hobby is making jewelry. She loves flower essences. She has been a healer for nearly thirty years.

I was showing Nina pictures from my life and I came upon photographs of Sarah Jane. "That's your daughter!" Nina exclaimed.

"No," I corrected her, "that is my brother's daughter."

A friend from another country just sent me an e-mail with a photograph of himself with his new son and wife. He was beaming, and there seemed to be a circle of love around them that spoke to the bond of love all of us have with each other as humans, going beyond countries, cultures, languages, or customs. Looking at that picture, I knew that nothing mattered as much to my friend as his son and his wife.

When we see the child within ourselves, we can look at ourselves with fresh eyes and see our innate innocence and wonder. When we see the babies in our families and in our culture, we renew our commitment to live our lives for something greater than ourselves.

Chapter 18. Hugs

"I can be of no real help to another unless I see that
the two of us are in this together."

—Gerald G. Jampolsky, M.D.

Another one of my favorite ways to open the heart
is by hugging. I like to hug almost everyone. When
you hug a person—with both of your hearts literally
touching, you can use kinesiology to demonstrate
how that strengthens both of you. If, on the other
hand, you hug but on the opposite side of the heart,
it doesn't feel quite right. It feels like you are actually
avoiding making a true connection.

The scientific research shows that the moment you
touch someone, whether with a hug or in hands-on
healing, a deeply connective act of the heart ensues.
When you hug someone, your stress hormones go
down, your immune system gets a boost, and your
feel-good brain chemicals go up.

Researchers with the department of psychiatry

at the University of North Carolina at Chapel Hill conducted a study of about 185 adults.[1] Group 1 consisted of 100 adults who were either married or with long-term partners. Group 2 consisted of eighty-five adults without their spouses or partners.

Group 1 was asked to hold hands while watching a ten-minute video, then hug for twenty seconds before giving a talk about a stressful experience. Group 2 was asked to rest quietly, then talk about a stressful experience. Following the brief speech, everyone had their blood pressure and heart rate analyzed.

After talking about something that really stressed them, everyone's blood pressure and heart rate went up. However, the rise in systolic blood pressure and heart rate was twice as high in those who had not given or received the hugs. It seems that even science can prove that hugging can offset our response to stress.

---

1 http://endeavors.unc.edu/win2004/hugs.html

CHAPTER 19. WHITE LIGHT

"To whatever degree you listen to and follow your intuition, you become a creative channel for the higher power of the universe."

—SHAKTI GAWAIN

Another way to open your heart is to visualize white light pouring through it. Although white light appears colorless, it contains the vibrations of the full spectrum of light and, therefore, includes the healing benefits of all colors in a balanced way. If you've ever seen white light going through a prism, you understand what I am talking about. White symbolizes purity and cleanliness. Channeling white light can connect us to the realm of spirit.

I invite you to participate in an exercise that will help you to open your heart. In a standing position, visualize white light coming in through the crown of your head. Allow the white light to pour first into your third eye, the energy center between your eyebrows. Then allow that white light to pour down into your heart.

Then, from the heart, allow the white light to pour down each leg, into the soles of each foot. And then allow the white light to flow from your heart out into each arm, into the palms of each hand. Visualize your whole being full of white light.

You can say a simple mantra while doing this:

I INVOKE THE LIGHT OF THE CHRIST WITHIN.

I AM A CLEAR AND PERFECT CHANNEL.

LOVE AND LIGHT ARE MY GUIDES.

As you see and feel the white light, feel yourself opening up your energy centers. Feel your heart open and relax. Feel yourself connected to your highest guidance.

Chapter 20. Affirmations

"A man is literally what he thinks."

—James Allen

You can also open your heart through your words. Your body believes every word that you say. How did you feel when you said the words in the last chapter? Were you able to feel the connection to your higher self, to your Christ-like self? Once you understand that connection, you can put your hand over your heart and feel the difference as you use specific affirmations. One of the simplest affirmations that I like to use is:

I HAVE NOTHING TO GIVE OR RECEIVE EXCEPT UNCONDITIONAL LOVE.

NOTHING COMES IN AND NOTHING GOES OUT EXCEPT UNCONDITIONAL LOVE.

This affirmation is also a great way to keep your energy protected. You can shut your eyes and visualize a bubble of energy around you. I like to put gold on the inside of the bubble and silver on the outside of the bubble.

As I do my visualization, I know I am divinely protected. I also like to affirm:

THE LIGHT OF GOD SURROUNDS ME.

THE LOVE OF GOD PROTECTS ME.

I AM A LIGHT OF GOD'S LOVE EVERYWHERE I
GO WITH EVERYONE I MEET.

CHAPTER 21. YOUR DEEPEST INTELLIGENCE

"All I know is that I do not know anything."

—SOCRATES

As we open our hearts, what we notice is that information starts opening up for us in an unfolding process, as if life were being revealed layer by layer. This kind of knowing from learning is different from the old way of studying like we did in school: measuring, adding and subtracting, reading or analyzing.

We get things on a deeper level. One of my favorite words to express this experience is grok: we *grok* people and events around us. To grok, according to Wikipedia, is a verb meaning to intimately and completely share the same reality or line of thinking with another physical or conceptual entity. Even if we don't call ourselves intuitive or think of ourselves as being intuitive, it just kind of happens.

If you look at an apple, for example, you might be able to see the surface features, notice the colors, and the shape and size. When you grok an apple, you can look at an apple and comprehend its taste, its weight, how it will feel in your hand, the age of that apple, and how long it will go without spoiling. You will know everything you need to know about that apple. You will get it at a deeper level, beyond all appearances and anything you could prove by any known scientific method.

Why is this the case? We know that when we synchronize our brain and heart activities, our heart and our brain come into entrainment. That is one answer. But I will give you another, simpler answer. When you love someone with no reservations, with no conditions, with no ifs, ands, or buts, you will know whatever it is that you need to know about them. It's just like the example of Gabe and his gardening: his love of plants, shrubs, and flowers expands his knowledge to the point that he knows just what to do to make them shine with radiance.

This is a state of being neutral, for sure, in that you are not projecting any negativity onto another person. Being neutral is absolutely essential to access psychic or intuitive information. You must be able to be in a neutral state yourself, where you are calm, grounded, and centered. Because we are all human, we can all go negative from time to time, and if you are feeling that way, you are not neutral.

This is one of the reasons why spiritual practices, such as meditation, yoga, or qi gong are so important in everyday life. They help us to calm down, relax, and be in tune with our higher spiritual energies. They help us to become neutral. When you see from this neutral state, you are seeing another person with the eyes of God, as God would see him or her. No matter how big of a mess the person appears to be in on this material, physical level, you realize that he or she is exactly where he or she is meant to be.

A mother who loves her child knows exactly what she needs. A father who loves his child knows exactly how to care for him.

Many left-brained people believe that all knowledge has to be acquired the hard way. You go to school. And schooling is good—I am all for that. I have a lot of left-brained education and find the world full of fascinating subjects.

You read books. And books are great. It is wonderful to assimilate the points of view of numerous authors.

You take classes and seminars as an adult to further your professional education.

And yet for all your degrees, all your learning, everything you have ever read in a book, there is no way to really know anybody unless you actually love them unconditionally. When you love someone or something unconditionally, you access your highest intelligence.

Chapter 22. Confusion about Love

"You are not here to sacrifice your joy or your life.
You are here to live, to be happy, and to love."

—Don Miguel Ruiz

About a year before I wrote this book, I had a major challenge to my views about love. One of my clients had been suffering from depression for about twenty-six years—ever since the birth of one of her children. She had damaged her feet from years of triathlons that were inadequately supported by her nutrition. She had two or three foot surgeries and had a screw in one toe. Another toe had damaged nerves. Her adrenal burnout was so severe she was tired pretty much all day long and didn't have the usual energy to do her exercises.

Before she met me, she had given up the thought of ever feeling better, mentally or physically. As we began to work together, her depression lifted. I used amino acids and supplements to balance her brain.

I did hands-on healing with her. I used kinesiology to balance her brain chemistry. I did deep emotional work with her to clear core issues.

Her foot pain went from a constant level of ten—on a one-to-ten scale—to days where her feet didn't hurt at all. She began to be able to feel there was hope for her case.

Her husband, however, kept questioning our work together. I offered to meet with him to explain what we were doing. The discussion immediately began with a question:

"Why did you send my wife an e-mail telling her, 'I love you, too?'" he demanded.

He let me know that during his years as a chief executive officer in charge of 1,000 employees, he had his adrenal function tested. He did not believe there was anything to it.

"I love my wife," he said to me. "You don't love my wife."

"I am sure if you asked any of her friends, they would all say they love her also," I responded.

"Care," he corrected me.

We looked at each other for a moment. It was obvious to each of us that on this point we would not agree. I explained that it was not uncommon for my clients and me to develop deep levels of trust, affection, understanding, and yes, love for each other.

"I have talked to a professional therapist, and she says it is not okay to tell someone you love them if they are paying you money," he insisted.

I thanked him for his point of view. I thanked him for coming in and speaking to me. He let me know that my services would no longer be needed—even though his wife had never done any therapy or taken any drugs before then that had healed her depression or alleviated the pain in her feet.

Even though he was a religious man, he did not seem to comprehend *agape*, the highest form of love expressed in the Bible. Although he himself had children, he did not agree that friends could experience *philia* for one another, and that when his wife's friends told her, "I love you," that they could actually be within social norms.

In the corporate world, it is not only unprofessional to express love to anyone, it is also foolish and could potentially open up a person to lawsuits. Similarly, in many therapies, healthy boundaries between client and practitioner may become blurred or confused. The purpose of these boundaries is actually to help create safety for all concerned.

In my experience as a healer, I have found that creating the space where people feel safe to be who they are and comfortable discussing what they are actually thinking and feeling can be the most transformational tool they have ever experienced. Often, a question I use when first working with a nervous client is, "What do you need to feel safe?"

The wife of the retired executive had felt safe enough with me to tell me all about what she had really been thinking and feeling. In so doing, she had begun to unburden herself emotionally, and the result was physical healing. We had talked about everything—her husband, children, dog, and her relationship with her body. However, her husband became threatened because his own definition of "love" was limited.

We have to remember that when we raise our level of consciousness, we become just that, more aware. We simply perceive a bigger picture. When we become more aware of what is actually going on, that includes compassion for those who have a little picture.

I kept myself totally together while listening to my client's husband. It seemed that, although he had made a large amount of money, he didn't have a very big picture about love. He also hadn't had the advantage of studying hormones or learning what is actually required to heal someone.

I used everything I had learned from all my years of spiritual study to listen to him, to allow him to feel right, to feel heard and respected. Then I fell apart and spent many hours crying! I questioned my mushy approach. Although I can appear quite strong, on the inside I am really a marshmallow and people who get close to me experience that. I have had to become strong enough to handle my sensitivity, but I am still quite sensitive.

Up to that point, I had ended all my letters and e-mails with "Love C." I sought the advice of other professional therapists about how best to communicate without creating the wrong impression. After that point, I concluded, "Love and light, Catherine." I wanted to make my intention clearer: to broadcast love and light from my heart in the way of *agape*, unconditional love—not to be mistaken for the personal.

Chapter 23. Love Is the Most Healing Force in the Entire Universe

"If you cannot find the truth right where you are,
where else do you expect to find it?"

—Dogen Zenji

Shortly after the incident with my client's husband, one of my friends was reading the sports news. He came upon a news story about a great assistant coach. The coach went above and beyond for all his football players, and the players knew what he was doing for them. "I love you, man," the coach was quoted as saying to one of his players. Even in the world of sports, or maybe even especially in the world of sports, the importance of love as a leading force is obvious to all concerned.

Although I have a huge menu of healing services, I have always felt that my secret weapon was my ability to love other people. All the other techniques that I know were to me just that, techniques. The real thing that gets things done, the real reason people got better when working with me, I have always felt, is love.

Why is this the case? It is a scientific fact that when two or more clocks are in a room together, they come into entrainment. That means they keep time together. When two or more people are within three feet of each other, their brain and their heart activities begin to synchronize. When you are in a state of love and appreciation, your own personal brain rhythms and heart rhythms, your EEG and your EKG, begin to come into harmony.

And when you are in a state of love and appreciation—even if it is just for your dog or the orchids in your studio, your late night dancing, your best friend, or even the sunrise you saw this morning—then other people have the opportunity to synchronize with your higher level of functioning. And when that happens, you are in entrainment and other people entrain to you. Then real healing happens.

CHAPTER 24. ENTRAINMENT AT A HIGHER LEVEL

"When you meet a swordsman, draw your sword:
Do not recite poetry to one who is not a poet."

—THOMAS CLEARY

When a group of women meet regularly, their menstrual cycles tend to coordinate. This is just another example of what I mean by entrainment. I remember when I used to have my period, my yoga students and I would all be walking up the steps to class groaning at the same time. When we are in a state of love and appreciation, that high frequency sets off a powerful attractor field that has the potential for great leadership.

In a field of unconditional love, anything can get better precisely because living tissue is alive, has frequency and vibration, and has the opportunity to synchronize to higher vibrational frequencies.

Illness is simply slowed-down vibration. You can understand what I am talking about because when you are sick, you feel heavy. When you are well and feeling healthy, you feel as light as a feather, efforts of all kinds are fun, and you even get ecstatically excited to challenge yourself.

So, understanding this:

- go for a walk
- hug your child
- write a poem
- do a dance
- take a nap if you are tired
- think a positive thought
- tell someone you love him or her
- say you are sorry
- let out a sigh
- cry until you are done crying
- laugh
- surround yourself with a beautiful environment
- walk in the woods
- smell a flower
- watch the sun rise
- pet your dog
- take a shower and enjoy the warm water flowing over your body
- appreciate the meal you are having, and give deep thanks for everyone and everything that went into making it

The general thought is that healing has to be difficult, expensive, or profound. Maybe it's as easy as simply learning how to shift your vibration to a higher level by learning to love and deeply appreciate the simplest experiences of your life.

Chapter 25. Connecting at A Higher Level

"The only real valuable thing is intuition."

—Albert Einstein

Many books about intuition talk about the psychic gifts, but nobody really talks about what turns on and what turns off your intuition. Intuition is simply connecting at a higher level. If you engage in judgment—a clear left-brained activity—that's the opposite of intuition. Judgment cuts off our connection.

How do you know if you are going into judgment? If you feel any negativity toward another person whatsoever, you are going into judgment about them. *A Course in Miracles* (ACIM International, 2005) teaches us that the world we see is merely a projection of our own mind. "Nothing I see in this room (on this street, from this window, in this place) means anything."[2]

The Bible says: "Judge not, that you be not judged" (Matthew 7:1). Also: "Judge not, and you will not be judged: condemn not, and you will not be condemned: forgive, and you will be forgiven" (Luke 6:37). So, to use our intuition, we actually have to bypass our own negativity.

Since each of us is still human, and we humans all have moments of grief, fear, sadness, pride, hate, craving, blame, shame, and other low-frequency emotions, then bypassing the sheer weight of all that can be quite challenging if we don't have ongoing stress management capabilities. To do intuitive work, you have to be relaxed within yourself. To do intuitive work well, you must not be stressed. And to do intuitive work at the very highest levels, you must not go into judgment about whatever it is that you see or hear, know or discover.

At a party I attended recently, someone mentioned that I had cleared the energy in the home where we were having the party. I had done the house clearing a few months beforehand as a gift to the host, Gerald Alvarez, who in turn had been a great friend to me during a particular challenging time in my life. The house was next to a Confederate battlefield and cemetery. In addition, he had bought the house in foreclosure from an owner whose business had failed. The house was renovated but the original structure was well over 100 years old. I wanted my friend Gerald and his new wife Ginger to be happy there, so I offered to do a house clearing.

2 Foundation for Inner Peace, *A Course in Miracles*, Workbook
  Lesson 1.

A lady there heard what I had done, and she came up to me with tears in her eyes.

A guy she had been dating had died suddenly in a motorcycle accident. She wanted to talk to me to understand what had happened. I don't usually like to do what I do at parties, not to mention not to make a big deal about it. But I saw that the lady was very upset, so we went to another room and sat down.

I saw the accident in my mind. A lady driving a van had hit her friend. The lady in the van dropped something and was reaching down to pick up something on the floor when she ran into him at a stop sign. His motorcycle was flipped up in the air and he died pretty much instantly.

The room where I was having this conversation was open, and another woman walked through. "Do me, do me!" she insisted.

I felt cornered and awkward, but I did not want to be rude. So when I was finished talking to the lady about the motorcycle accident, I went into yet another room where I had hoped I could be more private.

The second lady started asking me about her son. She actually had two sons, but there was one from whom she had been disconnected. I looked and saw and understood.

It wasn't a pretty picture, and it wasn't the sort of picture a mother would normally like to hear about a son.

Her estranged son had a business—if you could call it that—robbing people's houses in the middle of the night. He would get up about three or four in the morning and do his break-ins. Then he would sell the loot on the internet. Among the items he was stealing were guns. I told her that the government was onto him. She was understandably concerned about her children.

As I had only seen this lady once before in my life and knew nothing before then about any of her children, all this came as a surprise to me.

Gerald later confirmed to me what I had told the mother. "He is a thief," he told me, affirming that the son in question had once run up about $30,000 in bills on his mother's credit cards and that their relationship had been strained for years.

Paradoxically, I was able to receive this information because I had no judgment about it. Doing an intuitive reading is like reading the words on a page of a book without reacting negatively to what you read. And anyone seeking greater access to intuition would be wise to follow this program. Learning how to clear your mind of any judgment that might filter through is vitally important in understanding things on an intuitive level.

Chapter 26. Everyone Is on His or Her Own Spiritual Path

> "We can do more than just tap into the senses of
> other people. We can also tap into reality itself to
> gain information. As bizarre as this sounds, it is not so
> strange when one remembers that in a holographic
> universe, consciousness pervades all matter, and
> 'meaning' has an active presence in both the mental
> and physical worlds."
>
> —Michael Talbot

Even when I receive information that I would
rather not know about, I know that each of us is
on our spiritual path. Everyone has things that
have happened. Everyone can tap into the frailty of
humanity.

Some of us have done a lot of spiritual work.
Others have not yet started. Some of us have grown,
spiritually speaking. Others are still unconscious.
As we raise our level of consciousness, one way of
looking at it is that we are becoming more aware.

Some of us can look at the surface of an apple and get the picture. Others can really grok it. But no one is really better than anyone else. No one is really worse than anyone else. No one is really more important than anyone else. On a soul level, we are all the same. It is easier to love other people, I think, when we realize that.

As we become more aware, we are aware of how much our words, thoughts, and deeds affect other people—and not just other people, but indeed the entire world we live in. On the one hand, you can look at things as having a cause and an effect, but the truth is that everything that happens is subtly dependent on everything else that is happening. And that means that the true root causes, the exact and precise meaning of any event, is often greater than we can perceive. Simply put, it's a bigger picture.

Years ago, when I was first learning about my gifts, a woman told me that I have an angel that gives me the ability to tell someone the worst thing about them in the most delightful way. "That is true," I told her. "I can tell someone that they are a mass murderer and we can have a good laugh about it."

This was a bit of an overstatement, to say the least: I am thankful to report that I have not worked with any mass murderers. However, I do remember working with a man in England who had suffered from severe pain in his pelvis for many years. Because of the pain, he had received many injections and had become toxic from all the medication. He was holding the toxins in his joints and suffered from a lot of joint aches and fatigue, preventing him from doing much exercise. Even a simple walk could wear him out.

I remember during that first session explaining to him that it all went back to his younger years. He was a golf pro at the time and had enjoyed a very active sex life while he was single. In fact, he was so promiscuous that he would often have several partners in one day.

Looking at it, I couldn't figure out how he had managed to fit all that activity into his schedule. But he managed. I explained to my client that the pain in his pelvis went back to that time in his life.

He laughed. How did I know that, he wondered? But at a deeper level, he understood exactly what I was talking about. We have since worked together for many years. His pain is gone. His fatigue is gone. He has forgiven himself and developed a more balanced life. He has come to see that he also has intuitive abilities, and that during that particular time in his life when he was so active, he was in fact practicing his intuition to communicate with women without actually understanding what he was doing.

Chapter 27. Humankind Cannot Bear Very Much Reality

"If you bring forth what is within you, what you bring forth will save you. If you do not bring forth what is within you, what you do not bring forth will destroy you."

—Gospel of Thomas

When you begin to set aside your habit of constantly judging and see and are aware of more information, sometimes you get more data than maybe other people want to hear, even if they are paying you.

Once, a friend was very eager to develop her own intuitive abilities. She had been studying healing work while making a living as a marketing executive. She had a session with me to understand what she would be doing in the future. I told her that for the next several years, I saw her doing both healing work and marketing work. Unfortunately, she did not like this answer.

She asked a mutual friend who is gifted, and the mutual friend gave her the same insight. It didn't mean that anyone thought any less of her healing or coaching abilities. It was just what we saw.

Another friend endured a breakup after her boyfriend left her. She called me to ask what was next. "There is going to be a bit of a gap," I said as gently and carefully as I could.

"Oh no," she protested. She said she had all these guys lined up who wanted to date her. She would go out on one or two dates, but ended up turning them all down.

Another client had put her homestead on the market. She was eager to sell after an unexpected divorce. I didn't see her for a few months, then she e-mailed to invite me to lunch. She said she was upset that I had told her that it would not sell as quickly as she had hoped. I explained that I have to give the information spirit gives me, un-sugar coated.

Getting to neutral, being in a state of love and appreciation, doesn't mean that you get exactly what you want to hear. I think that one reason that many people do not fully access their own intuition is that they have all the information that they can currently handle. If we fully comprehend the implications of every choice we make, we might slow down and be more prayerful about every meaningful activity.

Chapter 28. Loving People You Have Never Met

"Viktor Schauberger, a pioneer in the movement of water, was known as 'the Water Wizard.' When asked how he developed his theories relating to the dynamics of the flow of water, he replied, 'Very simply, I have merged my consciousness with it.'"

—Emilie Conrad

If intuition is a byproduct of unconditional love, how do you go about loving people you have never met? Many people make the mistake of thinking you can only love people you know. Remember the story I shared in chapter 22. Love has nothing to do with knowledge in the way that most people think of it.

You can read all the books, get the degrees, be an accomplished expert, do the lab tests, weigh and measure precisely, and still not really know much about someone or something. Love is a quality of being in the world.

Some people talk about the kindness of strangers. You can often be kind to people you have never met because you don't have any history with them and, therefore, no issues. This is still not the power I am talking about. You can love people you don't know and have never met as a quality of heart. This quality is compassion.

To access compassion, you access the value of brotherhood/sisterhood. This comes close to the Greek word *philia*, but I think it goes beyond *philia* to comprehending the depth of our overall connection. The same molecules that I breathe out, you breathe in. The same earth I care for in my garden is the same earth that nurtures crops in China.

If I poison my garden with chemicals, or cheat someone at the grocery store, I create a chain of events that affects everyone. On the other hand, if I think through how I can raise my garden with the least damaging effect on the environment, and how I can be fair in all my dealings, that creates another ripple that comes back to me with kindness. In other words, whatever I put out, I receive.

I always feel the most selfish thing I could ever do is be kind, compassionate, and thoughtful to everyone. You and I may like the same baseball team. That helps.

Our sons may go to the same school. We could have grown up in the same state, voted for the same candidate, have to pay the same high tax rate, and drive the same roads to work. We may have the same reaction to the rain, shivering in the cold, or feel the same hunger at dinnertime. But compassion is way bigger than that. To be compassionate for others, we have to be welcoming of our entire experience as human beings.

I truly believe that we are all here to support one another, and that no man or woman is supposed to do it all by himself or herself. A simple way to access compassion is to see with the eye of your heart.

Chapter 29. Seeing with the Eye Of Your Heart

"Intuition is seeing with the soul."

—Dean Koontz

Even if you have never met another person, you can visualize him or her in the middle of your heart. Seeing with the eye of your heart is one of the simplest ways of awakening your intuition.

As you place that person in the middle of your heart, you can gain a tremendous amount of information about him or her.

- You can feel how he or she feels.
- You can see the way he or she looks.
- You can hear his or her soul speaking to you.
- You can know his or her struggles.

Because whatever air I breathe out you also breathe in, wherever you are in the world, we are all energetically connected. It's simply a matter of focus.

Place a person you don't know in your heart. This could be a person on the other side of the planet. It could be a soldier in a far-off war. Practice wishing that person health. Practice wishing that person happiness. Practice wishing that person safety. Practice wishing that person to be at peace.

Now you have accessed deep levels of compassion, and you will be the beneficiary. That is because as you access your compassion for another person, you will become calmer, you will become happier, and you will be able to know whatever it is that spirit wants you to know at this time. You will have aligned yourself with the vibration of unconditional love, a state that will awaken your highest intelligence.

Many of us are familiar with the concept of prayer. I myself have a prayer list at the back of my journal. This includes a list of everyone and everything I want to remember to pray about at the moment. I read over my list, think of each person on my list, and pray for their highest good.

It is my understanding and experience that because thoughts are actually things—literally vibrational patterns—when we pray, we are doing something quite powerful because we are sending our own energy out into the universe with the highest intentions.

Most of us, when we pray, have the habit of asking for something. Janis Joplin lampooned this idea with her song, "Mercedes Benz."

Oh, Lord, won't you buy me a Mercedes Benz?
My friends all drive Porsches; I must make amends.
Worked hard all my lifetime, no help from my
friends,
So, Lord, won't you buy me a Mercedes Benz?

Often, when we pray for someone, we think we
have a pretty good idea of what they need, even if
it isn't a Mercedes Benz. Maybe we think they need
healing or comfort or love. What we wish for ourselves
or another person may be very well intentioned and
perfectly reasonable. The other person may have
even asked for these things and asked us to pray on
his or her behalf.

Seeing with the eye of our heart is akin to a prayer
in that it is a spiritual practice. But, instead of asking
for things to be different, it allows us to perceive the
way things already are.

PART II:

PSYCHIC GIFTS AND THEIR APPLICATIONS

Chapter 30. The Gifts

"The intuitive recognition of the instant, thus reality...is the highest act of wisdom."

—D. T. Suzuki

As I have mentioned earlier, there are four primary psychic gifts:

- **Claircognizance:** the gift of prophetic knowing.
- **Clairaudience**: the gift of psychic hearing, also called intuition, but not to be confused with the general term. This is specifically hearing on another level.
- **Clairsentience:** the gift of psychic feeling.
- **Clairvoyance:** the gift of psychic vision.

Everyone has access to all these gifts, I do believe. Just as we all have eyes, ears, a mouth, and a nose, we can learn to access our ordinary senses and develop depth of perception with them through practice and training.

Whether or not you access your spiritual gifts has to do with many factors, but part of being able to access your extra senses is an understanding of how your gifts work. Many people are already using their divination in different places in their life without actually realizing that this is how they are accessing information. You can be a computer programmer, a Supreme Court judge, a traffic cop, a bus driver, a schoolteacher, or a veterinarian and be receiving this kind of information as a primary way of doing your work, making choices, and governing your life.

Even if you never plan to do intuitive readings for anyone else, if you understand your own gifts and how you may already be using them, you can come to greater inner peace. You will know you are being guided and protected every step of your way.

Just recently, I woke up early one morning and heard my angels speaking to me. "Remember when we kept the tree from falling on your house?" I heard. "And you think we would forget about you now?"

Sometimes it takes a rather dramatic event to remind us that we are being watched over. Even in the most mundane moments, your guidance is always there if you can only open yourself to receive it.

CHAPTER 31. CLAIRCOGNIZANCE: THE GIFT OF PROPHETIC KNOWING

"All minds are joined and are one."

—GERALD G. JAMPOLSKY, M.D.

The gift of claircognizance is the fastest gift to arrive. It is the best gift for getting advance information. It often gets information way ahead of time, so timing can be a bit of a problem. In fact, if you are a prophetic, you may receive information so much ahead of time, with absolutely zero corroborating information, that other people may question you or challenge you. Only later will everybody else catch up and see what you saw.

Just like you have physical eyes to see and physical ears to hear, you also have psychic centers where you receive information. The gift of claircognizance comes from above the crown of your head. Because it is the fastest gift, prophetic knowing often comes with no supporting evidence. That's the part that can be a bit challenging to other people, who are usually fishing for evidence to prove the validity of your information.

Only later, if you are prophetic, do you do a lab test to back up what you already know. Only later, if you are a prophetic, do things work out the way you had envisioned.

Because of my work as a health educator, I have worked with various laboratories for many years. It is helpful for my clients to have a lab test that they can then take to their regular medical doctor to back up what I have been saying.

I find that lab tests are often the best bridge between what I am explaining to my client and the medical doctor who has been treating them. That way we all have objective, quantified data that everyone can comprehend and agree upon.

Often, my propensity to make quick decisions—even about big, expensive choices—blows away people who are close to me. Once, I was looking to buy a house. I was flipping through a stack of black and white papers about real estate one Saturday evening. I came upon a one-page description of a house in the Collier Hills subdivision of Atlanta that I hadn't actually personally visited. I don't remember actually reading the page—I just saw the fuzzy photograph of the front door, which had a pot of geraniums next to it. I had no idea where the house actually was, had never visited the neighborhood, and didn't know anything else about it.

"That's my house," I said to my friend who was

looking through the papers with me.

"What do you mean, 'That's my house?'" my friend asked.

The next day, I went to the visit the house. I was inside for ten minutes and knew I needed to live there. The next day, an offer was in the works. That was a good thing because it had been on the market for less than a week and someone else was also making an offer. This is the house where I have now lived and worked for fourteen years. It is my favorite place in the universe and rarely a day goes by when I don't say out loud, "I absolutely love my home."

I am able to trust my guidance and make these kind of choices confidently because I have learned how my gift actually works. I am always explaining to my clients that if you have this gift, you will want to learn how to live with it so that you don't become totally overwhelmed.

Information will come barreling through like a freight train, feeling absolutely unstoppable. This guidance will interrupt all my other thoughts, probably making me appear distracted or a bit ODD. At other times, someone will ask me a question. All I have to do is focus on the person or place I am being asked about, just like setting a radio dial to a certain station, and the information comes rolling through without me having to do much else.

Because my brain seems to be processing much more energy than the average Joe, I like to live a very quiet life.

I am a prophetic. When I first learned about my gift, the lady who taught me about it told me that if it takes more than thirty seconds to get something, I am wrong.

Once I was scheduled to teach a weekend seminar in Seattle. Many people had signed up and had paid deposits to attend. However, every time I thought of actually going to Seattle on that particular weekend, I knew there was something wrong. So I ended up apologizing profusely and cancelling the workshop. This was months in advance—maybe four months before it was scheduled to begin. I questioned myself about this move, but every time I thought of flying into Seattle, I felt so uncomfortable, I knew I had made the right choice.

Finally, the weekend rolled closer. That Friday, Seattle experienced an earthquake that shut down the airport temporarily. I would have been flying in that day. I knew then that I had made the right choice.

Most people once again think of information as something you have to work for. The gift of claircognizance is the opposite of that. When you are prophetic, you get things very quickly and very easily. And, in fact, if you spend time mulling over things, that means your ego is getting in the way and you are likely to cloud the clarity of the directives you are receiving. Being prophetic makes you very good at being at the right place at the right time.

I will often know I am supposed to be at some place, and sign up before I know anything about it. I sign up for classes all the time, knowing I am supposed to be there to meet someone, make a special connection, or receive a special bit of information. Only later do I read the fine print.

Prophetics can therefore seem somewhat impulsive, but if you talk to a prophetic who is following his or her guidance, that directive will have felt like an imperative, like something very important that he or she just had to do.

This gift works perfectly if you want to show up at the right time for something as mundane as shopping. Although I am not a big shopper, I am always able to purchase things when they have been marked down 50 percent and I find a 15-percent-off coupon just that day. This makes the gift very practical if you want to go about saving money.

Once I was in a mall and saw a store I had never been inside of. I just knew I had to go in. It was the last day of a sale, and all the handbags were 50 percent off.

The good part about the advance timing of the prophetic gift is that it keeps you out of major messes that other people have not yet had time to pick up on.

Claircognizance can give you impressions of people to avoid, too. Years ago, the yoga community was abuzz with a man named John Friend, who had invented his own brand of yoga. He was featured in *The New York Times*, and it was very hip to say you were one of his certified teachers. One of the major mat manufacturers even hired him to brand one of its yoga mats. I saw John at a yoga conference at Kripalu Center for Yoga and Health once, and I remember thinking, *I don't want anything to do with him.* I did not know why. I just saw him across the room, very far away. Everybody else seemed to be looking up to him, thinking he was some kind of genius.

Flash forward at least ten years. He was only recently discovered to have stolen money from his company's pension fund, getting him in trouble with the U. S. Department of Labor. The fact that he had sex with a large number of his teachers and had gotten staff members to pick up his marijuana packages for him was the least of the scandals he had created.

I wondered if the yoga mat manufacturer had lost money because they did not have any intuitives on staff who could have had advance warning that they were making a bad investment. They had made a major investment in extralong yoga mats, which no longer bear his imprimatur.

Because the prophetic gift never shuts off and doesn't take time to figure out, you can learn to access this gift with no preparation.

Chapter 32. Clairaudience

"We can learn to accept direction from our inner, intuitive voice, which is our guide to knowing."

—Gerald G. Jampolsky, M.D.

Clairaudience has many aspects. It is literally reception of information as vibration. Vibration is often thought of as sound—it is—but it can actually be vibration, such as those experienced during earthquakes.

I used to have a client who had back troubles. I remember doing a healing to get to the root cause. It turned out he was an intuitive and was picking up on earthquakes in South America. Even for me, this was almost too weird. And yet he was very sensitive to vibration.

Clairaudience is often mistaken for your own thoughts because it can sometimes come to you in the form of words. I like this gift because it is very clear. "It's the foot," I will hear, when I am feeling a bit confused during my healing work.

Many writers and excellent speakers are using their gift of clairaudience. If you can remember chapter 11, where I was talking about "Amazing Grace," the author John Newton seemed to be inspired to write the words of the song. As you may also recall, these are the types of works that can resonate quite powerfully with an audience. These "inspired" artists are simply writing down or speaking the words they hear. This is also known as channeling, although many people who are channeling do not realize that they are actually doing it.

Once, I was sitting at a stoplight. I was second in a line of cars. The light turned green and the car ahead of me went through the intersection. I was ready to go, but I clearly heard the word, "Stop." I looked to the left. I looked to the right. I didn't see anything. The car ahead of me had already gone through. The light was green and, by all legal rights, I could move ahead. But I heard "Stop!" so I actually did. About that time, a car traveling about 60 miles per hour ran through the light on the other side. If I had been in the middle of the intersection, I would have been legally correct … but also dead.

Perhaps you can think of many instances in your life when you have heard a clear directive and followed it, only to save yourself or others. Or maybe you have heard the guidance but argued with yourself, only to regret not following your inner direction afterward.

We often use the gift of clairaudience when we think of a person and then they call us on the phone within five minutes of the thought. If you suddenly find yourself thinking of a friend you hadn't heard from in a while, that friend may either be talking about you or thinking of you at the same time.

When this happens to me, I will frequently pick up the phone or write a card. Once, I sent a pair of handmade citrine earrings to my friend Shirley Retter. She is the friend who taught me how to bead. When the earrings arrived, Shirley could hardly believe it, as she had moved to another city and we had not communicated in some time. She just had a minor medical procedure and was so glad to know that I had been thinking of her.

The center for psychic hearing is just above your ears on either side of your head. People who are highly attuned to psychic hearing are often very sensitive to noise. What may feel like an irritation to them may just be background sound to someone else. At the same time, these people make excellent musicians and sound technicians. One of my long-time clients, who is very proficient in this gift, runs a sound studio for movies, commercials, and soundtracks of all kinds. He can pick up the minutest change in pitch or tone.

What typically helps these people to rest is complete silence. When you are completely quiet, you can actually hear your guidance most easily. That's why meditation is so important, or why someone with this gift may do well getting up early in the morning or spending time late at night to listen carefully to the guidance he or she is receiving.

As we get better at differentiating what we hear as guidance from our ordinary thoughts, we can learn to listen to our guidance even in the midst of chaos. This form of guidance is usually very clear, positive, and direct. It is not muddled or worried, so if you find yourself ruminating or worrying, what you are hearing is actually your own ego and not your guidance.

CHAPTER 33. PSYCHIC FEELING

"This word 'intuition' is beautiful. You know the other word, 'tuition'; tuition means somebody else is giving it to you. Intuition means nobody is giving it to you; it is growing within yourself. And because it is not given to you by somebody else, it cannot be put into words."

—Osho

The center for psychic feeling, clairsentience, is in your solar plexus, just below your rib cage, the third chakra. There are a lot more feelers in the world than there are prophetics. That means that a lot more people use the psychic gift of clairsentience. The center for psychic feeling can make you a great people person, as you can intuitively pick up how other people are feeling. Most of my clients who are feelers are the sweetest, most considerate people you will ever meet.

Unlike prophetics and intuitives with psychic hearing, who are not knowingly bumble-headed about others but who often act and speak quickly without filtering the information they receive, feelers would never treat anyone unkindly; they can instantly feel other people's reactions to their words and deeds.

In fact, feelers often go out of their way to make other people feel good as that is the only way they can feel peaceful. They need everybody around them to be relaxed and happy so they can also feel relaxed and happy. Feelers often make great salesmen.

I had one feeler who told me, "Within ten minutes, I know how everyone in the room is feeling." The trouble with psychic feeling is that what you pick up is exactly that, a feeling.

Feelings come in all varieties. It can be a sensation of temperature. For example, I use my gift of psychic feeling to determine what to wear every day. I simply project my energy to wherever I am going to be that day and feel how hot or cold it will be.

In one day, for example, I knew to wear a light dress outdoors but slacks, a jacket, and a shawl to the play that night.

Feelings can also be emotions. When your emotions shift suddenly, what you are experiencing may not even be your own emotions. You could be feeling the emotions of your boss, your spouse, your child, or the person at the checkout counter.

Handling the gift of psychic feeling well requires a great deal of discernment. If you are not able to differentiate how you are actually feeling from any feelings you have picked up from others, you may end up feeling slightly loony or out of control, not understanding why you shift quickly from depression to glee. A good way to get better at using psychic feeling is to get by yourself three times a day and ask yourself how you are actually feeling. Then, if the feeling changes, you can ask yourself if you are picking up the energy of someone or something else.

This is a critical point for feelers to master. Once you become an expert at your own feelings, then you will become a true master at reading other people well. Until then, your experience of life may feel muddled and confused. The gift of clairsentience is what hands-on healers use to feel the health of your organs. (One of my friends, Shyamala Strack, is so talented in this area, she can feel the membranes in your brain!)

You can feel the energy not just of a person, but also of a place or a group. If you are trying to decide whether or not a group is right for you, for example, you can project your energy into that group and see how it will feel for you to be there. If you feel comfortable as you think of a group, you will more than likely feel that way when you get there. If you are uncomfortable, your own energy will contract, your breathing may be interrupted, and your muscles may tighten. That's a good indication of what you can expect.

If you project your energy ahead and realize that you will be going into an uncomfortable situation, you can ask yourself what you might need to do to shift the energy. Or maybe that is a very good sign that you don't need to go there at all.

Once my mentor in healing had planned to teach

a class. I adore learning and I am usually up for anything that will make me a better healer. However, whenever I thought about that class, I felt a very dark, heavy energy. I never signed up. It turned out that a few weeks before, she ended up having to cancel the class. Her mother had suddenly become ill and died six weeks later. It was a very traumatic time.

In the summer of 2005, I was visiting London. I was on a train going into the city and all of a sudden I felt this dramatic, overwhelming negative energy.

I am a Reiki master, so I drew the Reiki symbols in my hands, put my hands up and said a prayer to try to stop the incoming negativity. The energy kept coming and I was not able to stop it. I had never felt something like that before.

The next day I went to a crystal shop. I was immediately drawn to two aqua aura quartz crystals. I knew I needed to purchase them. When I got home, I looked up the healing properties of aqua aura quartz. They help with preventing psychic attack.

I was supposed to go into central London the following day. I went into the city and back with no problems. I was also supposed to go into the city the following day. However, every time I thought of going into the city that day, I knew I would have a very hard time coming back.

I debated with myself about this because a friend had scheduled for me to see ten clients in his studio. I called my friend and cancelled all the appointments. He was dumbfounded at first, as he had gone to great lengths for all these people to come and see me. I had to inconvenience not only my friend but also ten other people who had scheduled time out of their busy week to come and meet me.

I held firm. I was regretful, and apologized for inconveniencing everyone. The morning I was supposed to go into the city to see everyone, I had nothing to do, so I went for a walk for about an hour. I came back after my walk and saw the television in the house where I was staying. Four Islamic terrorists had blown up the subway, in three quick, successive bombings, and then a bus. The entire London subway system was thrown into chaos, and fifty-two people were killed.

I must have seemed very rude when I cancelled all those appointments, but after the bombs, I think everyone understood.

CHAPTER 34. CLAIRVOYANCE

"The third eye acts as a 'switch,' which can activate higher frequencies of the body of energy and thereby lead to higher states of consciousness. From a therapeutic point of view, it has been my experience over the years that many clients get better when they connect with their third eye, whatever the nature of their problem."

—SAMUEL SAGAN, M.D.

Everybody gets excited about clairvoyance because it can seem the most "real." I have numerous photographs of angels I have taken in and around my home and studio. You can see them at *www.catherinecarrigan.com*. I also have found angels in a field of sunflowers most recently, and they have shown up in videos that other people have taken of me.

How this happens, I honestly can't explain to you. I can only show you the pictures and you can decide for yourself.

Clairvoyance may give you a symbol. For example, recently I was in a church and a woman there said her daughter did not want her to have a relationship with her granddaughter. All of a sudden, I saw in my mind's eye a symbol. It was an equal sign with a slash through it, the "not equal" sign. I gathered they had never had an equal relationship. The trouble with symbols is you still have to figure out what they mean.

The gift of clairvoyance is also the gift you can use to see auras. You can train yourself to be able to do this. A simple way to do this is to relax your eyes and look past a person, as if you are looking for someone standing behind them. This is easiest to do if they are standing with a white wall behind them. As you relax your eyes and look past them, you may see evanescent colors, translucent light. You could also see the outline of their angel.

I had one client years ago whose aura I could see very clearly. She had fibromyalgia and chronic fatigue. Her aura was literally dark like the Peanuts character Pig Pen. She seemed to be carrying around a huge amount of psychic debris, which she experienced as pain and fatigue.

Once you understand that illness begins in your energy field, literally out there coming in toward the physical body, you will understand how important it is to keep your field clear. When your field is clear, it will literally look clear. There could even be light around your head.

One of the simplest ways to clear your field is by taking a bath with equal parts Epsom salts and baking soda. Qi gong also clears your field, as does walking in nature.

You can set your intention to clear your energy field every time you take a shower. Just visualize the water clearing not just your physical body but also your aura. While you are there, you can visualize your chakras, placing the correct color in each chakra so it will be healthy and energized.

When one of my friends came to visit, I could see her angel walking next to her as she walked through the door. It was just a flash, but I saw her angel. It was as if we were getting ready to have a happy get-together—my friend and I and all our angels.

When I look at the energy field of a person, I can see a lot of energies moving in different directions. Some people look very grounded while other people will have an energetic distortion. This is like walking through a house of mirrors. When you walk through a house of mirrors, you know your body is the same only it looks different depending on which mirror you are looking at.

I remember being at a meeting of art historians years ago. They all seemed to have big heads and little bodies. It wasn't true, of course. It was a slight distortion based on what was happening energetically. They obviously lived in their heads. Even though most of them were beautifully dressed, they paid little attention to their bodies.

An easy way to practice looking at a person's energy field is to watch a public speaker. I like to do this if I am going to church or a lecture, for example. The person is usually standing there long enough that if you pay attention, you will be able to tell what is going on. As you look and pay attention, what you may find is that energy is moving in unpredictable ways.

For example, during a recent church service, I watched as a church member led the public talk. I saw a diagonal arrow of energy moving from above her left ear down across her body. Meanwhile, her heart chakra seemed sunken into her body, and I knew she was protecting her heart.

Looking into the body is interesting as well. You can ask to see an organ and it will show you its shape, color, and size. One lady I saw had intermittent pain in her left lower abdomen. I was treating her with Reiki and, as I did my hands-on healing every week, it seemed her left ovary varied in size from week to week. At times, it appeared swollen. I encouraged her to talk to her doctors about it, but they could find nothing wrong. A month after I began treating her, she ended up in the emergency room. Her left ovary twisted and she was in terrible pain.

CHAPTER 35. A MÉLANGE OF GIFTS

"Whatever you do, even if you help somebody cross
the road, you do it to Jesus. Even if you give somebody
a glass of water, you do it to Jesus. Such a simple little
teaching, but it is so important."

— MOTHER THERESA

When you make a great soup, you may throw in
a whole array of vegetables on top of a healthy and
strong chicken broth, tossing in a bit of Celtic sea
salt and marinating the veggies in coconut oil. It's all
good and every ingredient matters. So it is when it
comes to using your own gifts.

More than likely, it will be easier for you to use one
gift better than the others. You can start by picking
the gift toward which you most naturally gravitate.
How do you know which is your easiest gift? You can
listen to your language.

You could say:

- "I know…" which would indicate you are using claircognizance.
- "I hear…" which would indicate you are using clairaudience.
- "I feel…" which would indicate clairsentience.
- "I see…" which would indicate clairvoyance.

I believe it's easiest to start with the gift you find most common to use because you won't have to work so hard. The harder you work, the more you are accessing your left brain and not using your gifts.

However, remember that it is important for you to be relaxed. If you are stressed, you will not be neutral. If you are projecting worry or any other negative emotions, you can't read what is actually there.

Even though I am highly gifted, I am equally gifted at knowing when I am not in a neutral state. Just like everybody else, I have my stuff! I ask other people for help when I can't get clear, or I wait until I am completely clear and then listen carefully. So often we want to hear a specific message when an even more important message may simply be, "No."

In retrospect, unanswered prayers can seem even more profound than the times when we get what we are asking for. Divine guidance is always on time and it is always correct. Everything else is the ego simply pushing and shoving and trying to control, not honoring the paths of our souls.

When you are asking for divine guidance, you can ask yourself what you know, hear, feel, and see. In this way, you may be able to gather a huge amount of qualitative information.

PART III:

MEDITATION:
ACCESS TO DIVINITY

Chapter 36. Start with Yourself

"At times you have to leave the city of your comfort and go into the wilderness of your intuition. What you'll discover will be wonderful. What you'll discover is yourself."

—Alan Alda

It is important that you start using your intuition with yourself. To use it wisely, you will want to begin by admitting you don't really know all that much, if anything—even on subjects you may have studied or practiced for many years—and are actually better off asking for guidance.

There are many reasons you will want to start with yourself. If you use your gifts too much for others and not enough for yourself, you will eventually become exhausted. That's because too much of your energy will be directed toward nurturing other people and not enough will be focused on helping yourself.

This will set up an energetic imbalance. We have

to keep putting cookies back into our own cookie jar if we want to be able to share with others. The second reason you want to start with yourself is because your gifts are the guidance from your soul. Your gifts are your soul actually speaking to you. If you do not listen to what your soul wants you to know, hear, feel, or see, you are missing out on important communication with your Higher Self. You are here to do you first. Only once you are doing you well will you be able to help others easily.

Let's face it: when you are not listening to your soul, you are blocked in the worst possible way. You are resisting what is. And you will not be following your path as precisely as you could be. Being blocked can show up in all kinds of unpleasant ways.

If you don't listen to your own soul, you can end up in the wrong job, the wrong marriage, you can end up in the middle of the intersection at the wrong time, on the subway in the midst of a terrorist attack, or you can miss the opportunity of your lifetime.

One of the best ways to learn how to tune into your own guidance is to start meditating regularly. Now I admit, it is only in recent years that I have gotten mildly good at meditating. I am too hyperactive, and have usually done better with meditative movement like yoga, tai chi, and qi gong.

I have learned more methods of meditation than I can even count, but the essence of meditation is finding stillness in the body so that the mind can clear. Often, when I begin to meditate, I see a picture of a pond. If you throw a pebble into a pond, ripples will flow out from the place where the pebble landed, but eventually the flow subsides and the wobbling stops. This is the picture I often see in my mind when the thoughts subside and I can begin to find silence inside myself.

The essence of meditation to me is being in the place where the ego mind can feel safe enough to take a rest. Quite simply, when we meditate, we feel at one with all that is. We experience our interconnectedness when the ego finally steps aside—even for a moment. That is when your soul guidance can come flowing through.

Many of us are so busy getting and spending that the thought of taking even five minutes just to be quiet sounds like a complete waste of time. In fact, the busier you are, the more important it is to meditate because your soul needs that open channel in order to communicate with you.

Sometimes people ask me if it's better to lie down or sit when meditating. The truth is, you can meditate while doing the dishes, going for a walk in the woods, or sitting quietly while petting your dog. There is no point at which anyone is going to anoint you with a wand and say, "You have got it! Good job!"

I sit in my meditation group, and you never really know what is going on inside anyone else. You just have your own experience.

Often what helps us to still our mind is performing a slow, calming movement, such as yoga, tai chi or qi gong. Our mind can be temporarily distracted by penetrating deep into the physical body, which has the paradoxical effect of freeing the soul.

If you wanted to start meditating for the first time,

I would recommend that you actually just lie down. If you were a little boy or girl learning to ride your bicycle, you might have training wheels. When you start meditating, give yourself all the training wheels you need.

Use an eye pillow to relax your eyes. Put a pillow under your knees. Throw a blanket over your whole body so that you feel completely comfortable and there is no physical resistance. Then just focus on relaxing everywhere you can think of relaxing. Close your eyes.

If you happen to fall asleep, it's okay; maybe you just needed more sleep.

Practicing daily in this way, you can begin to still your mind and find the restfulness inside.

Start with what actually works for you—whether it is sitting meditation, lying meditation, or meditative movement—and give yourself permission not to judge what that technique actually is.

Among the reasons that meditation is so important is that it creates a gap. Most of our lives are just jam-packed. We hustle from one activity to the other without pausing to feel, without taking a moment to look inside or ask for guidance about whether or not where we are going is actually in our highest, best interests. You have to have space in your life for this guidance to happen.

I surprised even myself when I discovered that I actually like to meditate. That is because I think that there are certain common themes that the soul actually enjoys. Our soul actually craves peace. Our soul craves order and beauty and love and companionship and time alone to process and fun and ways to grow in life. When you start giving your soul what it actually needs, you develop a better relationship with your spiritual self.

And, when you develop a better relationship with your spiritual self, you begin to start experiencing life the way your soul really experiences it, rather than the way your ego does: constant *sturm und drang*, pain and suffering, comments on attractions and aversions and what you think you like and what you think you don't like. This list goes on and on.

The benefits of meditation are legion. The benefits I have witnessed in myself and my clients include:

- Decreased anxiety
- Natural healing for depression
- Increased sense of happiness
- Better focus
- Improved immune response
- Faster healing of physical wounds
- Increased awareness of the oneness of all life
- Greater compassion for others
- Lower levels of cortisol and adrenalin, the stress hormones
- Higher levels of DHEA, the mother hormone
- Lower cholesterol levels
- Lower blood pressure
- Better quality sleep
- Improved ability to cope with whatever life brings

CHAPTER 37. THE GAP MEDITATION GIVES YOU

"The deeper you go in meditation your intuitive ability develops."

—SRI SRI RAVI SHANKAR

As you learn to practice meditation for whatever amount of time you can manage—five, eight, ten, twenty-five, or sixty minutes—you will start noticing that your energy feels clearer, and in this space of neutrality true insight and inspiration can drop in.

Having let go of your tragicomedy, even just for a non-commercial break in the action, the true experience of your soul begins to shine through. You start seeing with the eyes of your soul, knowing what your soul knows, hearing what your soul hears, and feeling what your soul feels.

This can be quite a bold departure from your usual course. In fact, you could feel like the old you died and you have been reborn again. This will be a good thing; it is from this quieter place that you can begin to use your intuition most effectively.

Although pain and suffering are integral to the experience of being human, it is in our moments of meditation when we achieve a right state of mind, a state of inner peace, from which true healing emerges naturally.

Chapter 38. Why I Like to Read For Health and Happiness

"There is more wisdom in your body than in your deepest philosophies."

—Friedrich Nietzsche

I told the story earlier about the woman who had asked about her son, who turned out to be a burglar. There's more to that story and, unfortunately, it doesn't end happily.

The story ended with the woman's other son committing suicide with the gun the burglar brother had given to him. The woman called me again, frantically, on a Saturday night, asking for help because she could not find her son. I beat around the bush; I did not want to be the one to tell her. I encouraged her to call her professional psychological counselor. I figured that would be enough of a clue.

Shortly after she called me, the police came to her

home to let her know they had found the body of her son lying in a cemetery. He had shot himself a few blocks from where his brother lived. It was a great tragedy for all concerned.

I choose to use my gifts to help other people be happier and healthier. In this way, I am using my gifts to be focused positively, a force for good in the world. We can all choose what to focus on. Even if I am looking at pain or suffering, I can use my gifts to look for a way to make things better. This is what I am about. You too can use your gifts to serve the light.

One of the best uses of anyone's gifts, I believe, is to learn to read the body so that you and others can experience higher levels of health and vitality. Because we all have a body, and we are always making choices about our body every day, I believe this is a very practical way to begin using intuition.

The body is also very concrete at a certain level; therefore, you can get immediate feedback when practicing your intuition. There are training programs that teach people how to do remote readings, but it would be much harder to hop on a plane to Afghanistan to find out if the mountain top you are reading is like you see it than it would be to start reading your own body, which is right here with you now.

In the next chapter I will explain to you how to do a simple body reading. I believe that your divine connection will strengthen and you can use your gifts in all areas of your life—to learn how to be in the right place at the right time, to know what you need to do to move forward spiritually, to live a more heart-centered and soul-fulfilling life.

Even though it is all God and, therefore, all good, I believe it is best to be focused on moving forward in life. And if what you are going through is particularly difficult, just keep moving and, eventually, it will probably get a bit easier.

CHAPTER 39. YOUR OVERALL LIFE ENERGY

"Knowing others is intelligence, knowing yourself is true wisdom. Mastering others is strength, mastering yourself is true power."

—LAO-TZU

One of the first things I look at when I am doing an intuitive reading for health is a person's overall life energy, chi, or prana, your vital force. You could call it your chi factor.

You can ask for guidance using a very simple number system, 1 to 100. The higher the number, the more radiant a person's life energy. The lower the number, the more a person is experiencing health problems and the lower their vitality will be.

Your chi factor is a total measure of your overall health, with the average for a person your age being around 50. What I have found is that when a number drops in the low 20s, that person is in a serious and possibly potentially fatal health situation.

Since nobody is perfect, and even those of us who are physically healthy also have mental, emotional, or spiritual challenges, I rarely if ever see anybody whose overall life energy number is in the nineties. A very good number is anywhere from 72 and over.

Fellow yoga teachers, tai chi and qi gong practitioners, regular exercisers, consistent meditators, healthy eaters, and people with low-stress lifestyles often have numbers in the 80s. This comes from years of being consistent and years of practicing activities that cultivate chi.

You can start on a health program and make improvements. But remember it takes seven years to make a whole new body. It would take about one month of detoxing for every year of really unhealthy behavior, such as excessive drinking or smoking. It takes about 120 days to build a new set of red blood cells, so if you start on a nutrition program, you would have to follow it for about four months to make a lasting change. So it takes time to build your health reserves.

If your number is really low, then I begin to look for deeper causes to find out what is depleting your chi.

Chapter 40. Your Will to Live

"The most powerful weapon on earth is the human
soul on fire."

—Ferdinand Foch

There is an energy point in your lower back
between your kidneys. When I am working with a
client, I check to see if his or her will to live is strong.
The point I use as an indicator for will to live is
called the Gate of Life. A person's will to live is an
indication that he or she wants to be here, that he or
she feels that life is worth living, that he or she finds
all the struggles and pains and suffering—grocery
shopping, visiting relatives, house cleaning, tax
paying, job working, and child rearing—are actually
worth it.

When a person's will to live is good, he or she will
do what it takes to get better. When a person's will
to live is off, he or she will often find conscious or
unconscious ways to check out, even if they appear

to others to be putting up a good fight. If your will to live is off, I will do a healing to release the root cause.

One of the root causes of lack of will to live is frequently deep levels of depression. My first book, *Healing Depression: A Holistic Guide* (Marlowe and Co., 1997), discussed the many ways you can overcome depression naturally. It was the best-selling book of the original publisher, Heartsfire Books, and went on to be translated into Chinese. It became the handbook for a network that was based in Seattle that taught people how to heal their depression naturally.

I do a tremendous amount of depression healing in my practice, and recommend a combination of therapeutic rest, emotional clearing work, and brain integration with kinesiology, amino acids, and other natural supplements to balance brain chemistry along with daily exercise. Even taking prescription antidepressant drugs may not alleviate the root cause of lack of will to live.

When you give up at the soul level, it may not be too long before you make a transition. I spoke openly about this to a friend whose cancer had returned. "What would it take for you to stay?" I asked. She told me a meandering story, but at the end admitted that if she did nothing the doctors said it would be sixty to ninety days. She passed just over two months later.

On the other hand, another friend told me about her mother, age 100. Even though the woman had been living in bed for years, she was determined to hang on. Family members would come over and crawl into bed with her, hugging her, begging her to stay. And so she did. Even when she finally passed, her death took many days and gave everyone in the family time to visit and time to say goodbye.

Resolving lack of will to live often means addressing deep psychological issues. I have never seen lack of will to live related to anything physical, even though lack of passion for living can have imminent physical effects.

Chapter 41. The Most Stressed Organ

"There is no such thing as a problem without a gift
for you in its hands. You seek problems because you
need their gifts."

—Richard Bach

The way I like to look at it, you can be a teacher
and have a great class of students.

But it's that one kid in the corner acting up who
drives everybody else crazy. If you can get that kid
to behave, then everybody else can settle down and
enjoy the experience.

Everybody has a "most stressed" organ, even very
healthy people. It's the organ you most have to look
out for now, or maybe even your whole life. The
cause could be a genetic weakness, stretching back
generations. Or it could be related to your soul's
experience.

For example, many souls choose to be born but
are not immediately successful at being incarnated.

When they are finally born, their actual birth parents may be their eighth, ninth, or tenth try, or so on. The emotions about that experience will affect an organ and possibly cause a lifelong weakness in that organ if it is not properly addressed.

For example, you could be angry that you ended up with a certain set of birth parents, and that anger could be causing a long-term weakness in your liver.

Your most stressed organ may affect your metabolism. For example, if your pancreas is constantly stressed from low self-esteem, you may appear physically huge, have trouble metabolizing sugar, and struggle with your body weight.

You can do a simple intuitive reading on the health of all the body organs using a number system that I mentioned earlier. The organ with the lowest number will probably be the most stressed organ.

When you find a person's most stressed organ, you can then uncover, on all the levels, what that person will need to do to be healthier in the long term. You simply ask the organ what it needs. So, for example, if your liver is your most stressed organ, on the soul level, you may need to practice forgiveness, to express your creativity, or to find out what makes you really happy. On the mental level, you may need affirmations about being a happy, vital, and strong. On the emotional level, you may need to find productive ways to release your anger. On the energetic level, you may need more exercise to release congested energy. On the physical level, you may need bitter herbs, more green vegetables, juicing, beets, apples, lemons, or a detoxification program.

Find a health professional who can do critical point analysis to identify which healing methods will be most effective for you.

If you take care of your most stressed organ, you can resolve root issues that may have plagued you your entire life and end up adding years and quality to your experiences.

CHAPTER 42. READING THE ORGANS

"Understand that you are a soul with a physical body (not a physical body with a soul) a spiritual being—energy—and that soul is the energy or the life force that keeps the cells of your body alive. If you are having trouble with your body, you need to go to your soul and see where you are going against your soul's plan in this lifetime."

—ANNETTE NOONTIL

I have already discussed a simple way to read the organs by asking the body for a number that indicates its overall level of functioning. We have established that a good, "healthy" number would be between 72 to 85. If an organ is under-functioning, once again you can simply ask the body and also ask the organ what it needs to begin to work better.

Although I have plenty of clients who are chronic overachievers, if an organ is overworking, indicated by a number higher than 85, that may mean that it is overcompensating for something else. For example, your adrenals could be overworking due to unrelenting stress. Or your brain could be overworking when you stay late at your job or continue doing business into the evening hours when you should be resting.

I am a big fan of healing with nutrition, so I generally start with healthier eating and move on to dietary supplements. I realize that other medical intuitives may feel that it is possible to be healthy and happy while eating a fast food diet. However, that is not my experience!

Healthy people generally are doing something to maintain their health, just as rich people usually carefully monitor their business and investments.

The way I use supplements is different. Most people research something on the internet but do not bother to find out if that supplement actually agrees with their bodies.

I like to use kinesiology for supplement testing. To me, kinesiology beats lab tests for this, and it also beats even electroacupuncture (EAV) machines that determine what a person needs but not whether the supplements recommended actually agree with that person's body—or, in fact, are working to make that person better.

Many nutritionists follow general protocols but are overloading their clients with supplements that the body can't process or assimilate. I also follow general protocols but take the process one step further by asking whether or not the supplement can be assimilated and tolerated. I also test to see how the supplement affects a person's blood sugar and hormone balance, and then, if it passes all those other tests, how it affects the organ it is supposed to improve.

You would be shocked to see how many people are wasting money on supplements that not only don't work, but that are actually making them worse. The supplements are either toxic or they can't be digested or assimilated.

Often one of the first things I do with new clients is weed out the supplements they are currently taking that actually make things worse. This saves them money and allows them to get better faster.

The very same question needs to be asked about medically prescribed drugs. I recommend everyone look up the side effects of all their medications. If you need to change a drug, ask your doctor.

I always say there are 100 ways to skin a cat. If you get stuck in a mental rut, I recommend that you write down twenty different ways you could solve your problem that do not involve medication. Then ask yourself if there is even one of those methods that you might be willing to try in addition to your drugs or instead of your drugs.

CHAPTER 43. BODY SYSTEMS

"In retrospect, it should have been obvious to me and to other biologists that Newtonian physics, as elegant and reassuring as it is to hyper-rational scientists, cannot offer the whole truth about the human body, let alone the Universe."

—BRUCE LIPTON

There are multiple systems in the body. These include your:

- Electromagnetic system
- Musculoskeletal system
- Endocrine system
- Nervous system
- Cerebrospinal fluid
- DNA
- Hepatic system
- Respiratory system
- Immune system
- Vestibular system

- Circulatory system
- Digestive system
- Genitourinary system
- Reproductive system
- Neurotransmitter system

Body systems include groups of organs that work together. Just like finding your most stressed organ, it is often helpful to find your most stressed system. You can ask the body to rank each organ system on a scale of 1 to 100. A healthy organ system will be operating around 72 to 85. If a system is operating at a low level, you can use your intuition to ask what the body needs to operate more efficiently.

So, for example, if your most stressed system is your digestion, which is very common, you will want to get to the root cause. The root cause could be low stomach acid. It could be a bad bacteria in the stomach, such as *helicobater pylori*. It could be low pancreatic enzymes, making it harder for you to digest your food fully. It could be poor assimilation in the small intestine, poor elimination in the large intestine, overall inflammation, parasites, or food sensitivities.

The digestive system is often the most important organ system to heal first. That is because when you heal your digestion, you eliminate inflammation that is the root cause of joint pain elsewhere in your body.

You can heal or eliminate food sensitivities that may be affecting your brain chemistry, since over 90 percent of serotonin is produced in your gastrointestinal tract, and you can finally digest and absorb the nutrients from your food, making it less likely that you will need a high level of nutritional supplements.

When you heal your digestive system, all your other organ systems can finally heal because you can get what you need to improve.

When I find a client's most stressed organ system, I figure out what is causing the organs in the system not to work well together. Sometimes the body just gets confused. Sometimes there is an emotional pattern that the client is holding that is keeping him or her in a state of distress. And, once again, I ask what it will take for that organ system to function at a higher level.

CHAPTER 44. ENVIRONMENT AND FENG SHUI

"The cell's operations are primarily molded by its interaction with the environment, not by its genetic code."

—BRUCE LIPTON

Many medical intuitives look at the body alone, not taking into account a person's environment. To me, this is a major mistake. Just like you can't take a beautiful orchid and put it in a dark room and expect it to thrive, you can't put an individual in the wrong place for that person and expect him or her to do well. To me, environment includes the physical setting.

This approach to healthy environmental living also includes the energy of your home, which experts call your feng shui. Feng shui is a Chinese system of geomancy using the laws of heaven and earth to improve your well being on all levels. But it goes beyond all that because some people need to live in a desert, others need a more active city life, while others thrive on a more peripatetic experience, traveling from place to place.

One of the more dramatic cases I can relate has to do with a young man who had been sick the entire twenty years of his young life. He had been everywhere: doctors, shamans, homeopaths, a mental hospital, psychologists, psychiatrists, chiropractors—you name it. He was so sick when he came to me he had trouble walking up the few back stairs to my studio. His spine was twisted and, even though he would visit a chiropractor, he would lose his adjustment as soon as he got home. He was so sick and exhausted he had not been able to complete school.

The story about how he got to me was an interesting one. One day, he was standing in his front yard, staring up at the sky. He said, "Dear God, please help me!" A few seconds later, the cell phone he had been holding in his hand rang. It was a feng shui practitioner.

Figuring it must be divine guidance, he called the practitioner to his home. She took one look and said to him, "You need to go to see Catherine." So he and his mother ended up at my studio.

His mother was almost as stressed as he was; she had devoted her entire life to trying to help him get well. She had recently quit her job in order to help him, which ended up being a blessing—he was unable to drive himself to our appointments. During our very first session, I told him, "Sixty-five percent of what is wrong with you is your environment." He had a terrible mold infestation in his home and was severely allergic to mold.

I helped him and his mother locate the best company to clean out the mold in their home. Years ago, their house had nearly burned to the ground. The fire department came and hosed down the house with water. What ended up being left quickly grew into mold in the Georgia heat. Any environment where the relative humidity is higher than 50 percent has the potential to become a haven for mold.

But that wasn't all of his environmental problems. I figured out that years ago there had been actual executions on the property. Numerous criminals had been put to death in their front yard. We discussed ways to clear the energy of those departed spirits.

As if all that was not bad enough, his father had passed away in the living room. The father's soul was hanging around to try to protect the son. The place was an environmental wreck, not just physically but also spiritually.

As we worked together to clear the environmental problems, my client's physical health improved dramatically. He ended up being able to walk eight miles a day.

Even gorgeous homes may have mold. I had a client who was an interior decorator who had problems with itchy eyes that no doctor had been able to relieve. I recommended that she test her home for mold. Even though I knew it was decorated to the highest standards, it still wasn't a healthy environment.

I like to refer clients to a classical feng shui

practitioner if I feel that the energy in their home is not right. Once you declutter, you can take things to a whole new level if you work with classical feng shui principles. Classical feng shui practitioners use a compass, and I find are far more accurate and effective in their approach than those who use other feng shui systems.

Another factor in your environment may be an overexposure to electromagnetic fields. One gentleman with whom I worked had high blood pressure. When I got to the root cause, it was his bedroom. He slept with his head next to an electrical socket. He had a TV and computer also next to his bed, which was an electric hospital bed that could be moved up and down with a remote control.

Your heart is electrical. Your brain is electrical. Your entire acupuncture system reacts to electrical impulses in your environment. You can balance your electrical system more easily if the environment you live and work in is clear and healthy.

Chapter 45. Rhythm

"Everything in the universe has a rhythm, everything dances."

—Maya Angelou

Rhythm is an unheralded and often overlooked aspect of being healthy. You can use your intuition to detect the rhythm of anything. Putting your hands on an organ, you can feel its rhythm. Projecting your energy into the New York subway system, you can feel that rhythm.

For example, most women know that a healthy female cycle averages about twenty-eight days, but there are many other natural rhythms in the body that can become dysfunctional when living against one's own natural harmony.

What is less well known is that every three hours, the energy in your body naturally shifts from one acupuncture meridian to another. In a twenty-four-hour cycle, the energy will have shifted through all the meridians. One of the most common ways to disrupt your body rhythms is with shift work.

I feel great compassion for people who have to work in the middle of the night. Working in bright lights when your body wants to be sleeping throws off your insulin balance, your brain chemistry, and all your sex hormones. You can lose weight, overcome depression, restore your energy, and balance your blood sugar just by finding a job where you can work during the day and sleep at night.

Sometimes rhythm is trickier than that. One of my clients works with horses.

I told her years ago that she really needed to be outside, working in direct sunlight; I was able to determine that her pineal gland was her most stressed organ. She had already intuitively understood this, having created a career for herself caring for horses. As earthy as she was, however, her soul longed for travel.

Ultimately, we figured the healthiest rhythm for her at the moment was for her to work two weeks on, travel two weeks off. She became happier and her soul felt freer because she was not being tied down to a traditional schedule.

You will know you are living at a healthy rhythm for you when your energy is consistently good, your mood is regularly happy, and you feel vital and productive. Many people do not do well on a nine-to-five schedule.

Eventually, the stress of having to live up to someone else's rhythm wears a person down. This may show up in mental/emotional problems or physical fatigue.

One of the key factors behind rhythm is how much your body needs to sleep and what time you need to go to sleep and get up. Every minute of sleep before midnight is worth ten minutes of sleep after midnight.

Rhythm can show up also in how often it's best for you to exercise. You can overdo even good things, exercise being one of them. If your sleeping rhythm is off, your exercise rhythm will probably be off as well; you won't be able to tolerate as much intensity on an ongoing basis. At the end of the day, it's all about finding what works best for you and your body.

Major life changes may require major adjustments to your rhythm. You may get less sleep with a new baby, for example, but that will mean you would need to cut back in other areas. During menopause, your adrenal glands may not allow you to push like you once did, and you may find yourself needing more rest than you did earlier in your life, even if you are healthy.

CHAPTER 46. OVERALL TOXICITY LEVEL

"There are so many unseen negative influences on human health that are missed by conventional medical practitioners that many sources of human suffering remain undetected. Disease susceptibility as a consequence of exposure to environmental pollutants is partly a function of the strength of the body's immunologic, physiologic and energetic defense mechanisms. Conventional safety limits of exposure do not take into account the subtle vibrational effects of toxic substances."

—RICHARD GERBER, M.D.

Two hundred years ago, toxicity wasn't as big of a problem as it is today. Over 70,000 new chemicals have been introduced into production and released into the environment in the past 100 years. Just as we can have environmental challenges like mold, or environmental allergies like sensitivity to ragweed, we can also have internal toxins.

Just as you did with organs and organ systems,

you can do an intuitive reading using a number scale, 0 to 100, to ask for toxicity level. In this case, the lower the number, the better. If you find high levels of toxicity, you can ask the body what the source of toxicity is. It could be heavy metals, chemicals, foods, or environmental sources.

Once you find the source, it will be important to find the organs being affected. This could most commonly be the brain, kidneys, and liver, but toxins can literally be held in any organ.

I recently did a lab test with a client who had been complaining of fatigue. I like to back up my medical intuitive readings with lab tests when resources permit because some things that are bothering you may not be that obvious. It turned out she had high levels of a paint solvent at the cellular level.

Her very first job out of college had been at a printing company. Although she exercised regularly, had a great marriage, and worked at a job she loved, she was actually not healthy because her body was not able to eliminate the chemicals she had absorbed virtually twenty-five years before. We worked together to detoxify the old chemicals and she felt better mentally, emotionally, and physically.

I like to check overall toxicity level and, when appropriate, encourage clients to detoxify. I have had so many clients with cancer. To me, it is a great tragedy when serious disease could have been prevented with simple lifestyle steps.

A great place to begin is with your diet. That is because you may or may not be able to control the chemicals you are exposed to in your environment, but you can control what you ingest with your food. Eliminate artificial sweeteners and additives, including aspartame and MSG. Choose organic produce when possible and hormone- and antibiotic-free meats and dairy products. Include as much fresh food like fruits and vegetables in your diet, as these have more life energy than heavily processed products.

If you were to see the energy field around toxic food and the energy field around fresh food, it would be a lot easier for you to make the right choice. You would run, not walk, in the other direction! You can put your hands over your food and if you are highly trained or sensitive with your hands, you can feel more chi in healthier food.

If you are holding toxins in your body, common signs are fatigue, brain fog, depression, or joint pain. Fat cells try to protect your internal organs from toxicity, so detoxing may go a long way to helping your body eliminate the body fat you may not have been able to shed via conventional methods. Eliminating heavy metals and other toxins can be done very easily through the use of a far-infrared sauna. I highly recommend far-infrared saunas for this purpose.

As you lower your overall toxicity level, you have the side benefit of clearing your aura. You will be amazed how, as your physical body and energy body clear, you will end up being more naturally intuitive.

I had already done more detoxing than anybody I knew when I got my far-infrared sauna back in 2004. I was amazed after using it and my energy level doubled. My intuitive gifts came through more clearly and easily as my entire body lightened up.

Chapter 47. The Body Levels

"Joyful cooperation with the 'God-in-everything' is the best medicine for all ills, the best way to achieve personal fulfillment. To do this, however, takes a commitment to remind yourself constantly of the presence of God in all people, places, things, and situations."

—Serge King

As you practice using your psychic gifts to begin reading the physical body, you may begin to recognize that there is more to the body beyond just the physical. Most people are aware of their physical body but have very little consciousness about the other levels of their body.

Your energy body includes your chakras, your breath, and your acupuncture system. Your emotional body includes all your emotions. (This is actually the most important part of you, as emotional problems can shut down literally any organ system, any part of your energy body, your mind, and even affect your soul's experience.) The mind level is the root of your beliefs. The soul level is the causal level, what you came in with, and what is going on with you spiritually.

These five levels together comprise your energy body, or aura. For healthy persons the aura generally extends about eight feet in diameter. For someone who practices energy work, such as a yoga practitioner, or a tai chi or qi gong master, an aura may be about 100 feet in diameter.

I like to get a sense of how big someone's energy field actually is. Anything within three feet of you will affect your total wellbeing because anything within three feet is inside your energy field. Having an electric clock, computer, or cell phone right beside your head at night, for example, may be a hidden cause of heart arrhythmia or insomnia.

The bigger your energy field, the more sensitive you may be to everyone and everything around you. If you have an expanded energy field, you will want to practice being grounded and centered. If you are a very sensitive person, you have to become strong enough to handle your own experience.

As you read the physical body, you can also begin to get a sense of what is going on with these other levels, and that will indicate to you what really needs to happen for deeper levels of healing.

PART IV:

HEALING

CHAPTER 48. THE FIVE LEVELS OF HEALING

"Healing does not mean going back to the way things were before, but rather allowing what is now to move us closer to God."

—RAM DASS

No matter what is going on with you—a sore thumb, broken toe, ripped rotator cuff, the flu, cancer—everything is always happening all the time on all five levels: physical, energetic, emotional, mental, and spiritual. If everything is always happening on these levels all the time, then in order to get truly well, you will want to look at what is going on at each level of the body and heal from all five levels.

One of the reasons that I am particularly effective as a healer is that I am able to deal with all five levels. I figure out which level is holding the dysfunction or imbalance, and then I clear it on that level. Most forms of healing only work on only one of those levels and leave out or ignore the rest. This, I feel, is a major mistake. You are a whole person.

To leave out even one aspect of what is going on with you is to leave out your chances for total and complete healing, or set the stage for your disease to return or morph into another form of dysfunction on another level.

Physical Healing

Most of us are at least somewhat aware of what physical healing might entail. Physical healing addresses the bones, muscles, organ systems, and a person's nutrition or exercise program. This might include tasks performed by a chiropractor, massage therapist, traditional medical doctor, nutritionist, physical therapist, or an exercise professional.

Energetic Healing

Energy healing entails any and all therapies that balance the energy systems of the body. This could include acupuncture, hands-on healing, tai chi, yoga and qi gong, Reiki, breath work, or healing touch. It could include rebuilding your chakras or repairing your hara line—the main vertical current of energy— or restoring all levels of your energy field.

Emotional Healing

Emotional healing may include visiting a psychologist, psychiatrist or traditional counselor, or any other therapies that help you get in touch with your feelings. I use kinesiology to clear emotions, finding where you are holding your emotions in the body.

Mental Healing

Mental healing may include any therapies that address your core beliefs. This could include EFT, Psy-K, Brain Gym, or using affirmations to retrain your thought patterns.

Traditional psychotherapy or working with a professional counselor may also empower you to re-examine mental patterns that had you running on automatic.

Spiritual Healing

Spiritual healing may include working on past life issues; karmic clearing; prayer; meditation; working with angels, guides, and power animals; color and gemstone therapy; invocations; learning how to protect and ground your energies; and the use of symbols such as a cross.

CHAPTER 49. WHERE DID IT ALL BEGIN?

"Your body tells you what you need to learn—it is your barometer."

—ANNETTE NOONTIL

It is important to realize that disease or illness of any kind begins in the energy field—literally out there—and comes into the physical body. That means that, more than likely, whatever you are suffering from physically did not actually begin on the physical level. When you are reading the body levels, you have to ask where a disease or illness actually began.

More than likely, whatever you are experiencing began on the energetic, emotional, mental, or spiritual level before condensing on the denser level of your physical body.

As I mentioned earlier, there is a flow of energy in the body. Energy comes in through the hara line, a vertical electrical current stretching from above the crown of your head to below your feet. The hara line feeds your chakras. I have gone into some detail about the seven primary chakras and many minor chakras. The chakras are energy plexuses that correspond to your major endocrine glands.

The chakras feed your acupuncture meridians. You have twelve primary acupuncture meridians that correspond to the five elements (fire, earth, metal, water, wood) and also to yin and yang polarities.

The acupuncture meridians feed your organs. You have seventy-eight organs in your body.

Your organs feed energy to your muscles. There are between 656 and 850 muscles in your body, depending on how you count them!

So, when we are feeling something in the way of pain and disease, we have to go back and rediscover where the original disturbance began. If you go back and go back and go back, you can finally discover the core issue.

CHAPTER 50. THE CORE ISSUE

"The doctor should be opaque to his patients, and like a mirror, should show them nothing but what is shown to him."

—SIGMUND FREUD

The core issue is the root cause. It could be simple, such as a thought you had: "I have had it. I don't want to put up with this mess. I don't want to be here anymore." Or it could be something more complex, such as the relationship you have had for years with your father.

For simplicity's sake, let's say that the core issue is either:

1. **Emotional**—such as a feeling you had or are still going through
2. **Mental**—a thought, such as an erroneous belief
3. **Fear-based**—which I put into a separate category because fears include both thoughts

and emotions

4. **Spiritual**—such as hesitation at the moment of your incarnation, or an idea that is wounding your soul, such as that you are not good enough or don't deserve the best in life.

Again, identifying the root cause, which will be on one of the physical, energetic, emotional, mental, or spiritual levels—very rarely on the physical level itself—is vitally important. It's always about YOU.

Identifying and rooting out the core issue is key to facilitating your total and complete healing. If you are reading the body, you will want to use your psychic gifts to ascertain the core issue. If you simply address symptoms, you could be chasing the tail of the dragon for many, many years.

Chapter 51. Are You Willing to Heal?

"What we experience is our state of mind projected outward. If our state of mind is one of wellbeing, love, and peace, that is what we will project and therefore experience. If our state of mind is one filled with doubt, fear, and concern about illness, we will project this state outward, and it will therefore be our experiential reality."

—Gerald G. Jampolsky, M.D.

In the initial assessment stages, one of the most important things I ever do is check to see whether or not a client is willing to heal. If I have a client who has been sick for a long time, this is one of the most important things I will ever check. If you are reading the body, you must check to see if a person is willing, ready, and able to heal or his or her unconscious self will block any attempts at serious progress.

The average client who comes to see me has already been to the medical doctor (even the Mayo Clinic), the energy healer, the psychologist, psychiatrist and mental hospital, the physical therapist, chiropractor, nutritionist, marriage counselor, etc. I am not better than any of these professions; I view all these professions as important and necessary.

But what is unique about my approach and what I find is important as we move forward as a global community, where resources for health are increasingly limited, is to work holistically and get to the root causes and eliminate them. Anything less is just fluffing the pillows or making a show of effort, rather than a complete change.

Willingness to heal is one of the most important aspects. When you are willing to get better, you will do whatever it takes. If you are not willing to heal, then no one can make a lasting difference.

This is where kinesiology comes in. You can also use your psychic gifts to ask the same questions. Try asking yourself:

- Am I willing to heal?
- Am I willing to benefit from healing?
- Am I willing to allow the changes to take place?
- Am I willing to act on what is discovered?

Your blocks to being willing, once again, may be:
- Physical
- Energetic
- Emotional
- Mental
- Spiritual
- Social
- Known
- Financial

Or they may be on some other level that is currently unknown to you at this time.

If there is a block to willingness, it is probably best to do a complete healing on that issue alone. Often, if you clear your blocks to willingness, that one step will allow you to make a major leap forward, both in your spiritual growth and your personal healing.

Chapter 52. Pain Addiction

"I make friends with hindrances and every obstacle becomes a stepping stone. Every-thing in the Universe, visible and invisible, is working to bring to me my own."

—Florence Scovel Shinn

Many people are unwilling to heal because they have grown addicted to their own pain. Believe it or not, you can be addicted to anything—not just food, sex, or rock 'n' roll. If someone is experiencing pain and you are reading his or her body, you will want to ask if the person is addicted to pain.

Pain addictions include:

- *An addiction to the idea that you are so special other people can get better, but you can't.* These are the people who find a reason to believe that while other people may have suffered from their affliction and overcome it, they have so many special circumstances in their lives that they can't.

- *An addiction to failure.* You will see a repeated experience of failure in multiple aspects of a person's life. If this is the case, work on self-esteem, self-identity, or self-efficacy issues. The problems may seem out there, but are actually within.
- *An addiction to drugs, legal or illegal.* Many people have been on so many drugs for decades that they don't know what their life experience would be like without them. An interesting exercise is to ask yourself and your doctor whether or not you still need the medication you have been taking.
- *An addiction to going from one doctor/therapist to another.* I have had clients visit as many as thirty different medical professionals with no improvement because the problem wasn't one that a medical professional could actually solve.
- *An addiction to isolation and refusing to participate in normal social life.* Illness can be an excuse to avoid going out into the world.
- *An addiction to avoiding sex and intimacy.* Disease can be used as a barrier to keep other people from getting too close.
- *An addiction to pessimism.* A negative outlook inside can be projected outward onto the world, as if nothing can ever get any better.
- *An addiction to withdrawal and escape.* It may seem safer in the small world of a person's comfort zone.

- *An addiction to depression, worry, or anxiety.* Many people are so addicted to these states of mind that they find a way to recreate new reasons for feeling bad. This attitude may get projected out onto the world or other people when the problem is actually due to personal patterns of thinking and experiencing.
- *An addiction to living in pain and suffering.* If you think of life as a game, you can learn how to actually be happy. We think it is our circumstances that need to be changed, but it is often our relationship with ourselves and the world around us that makes a bigger difference.

Underlying these pain addictions are payoffs. Payoffs are what you get by staying sick and in pain.

CHAPTER 53. PAYOFFS

"It isn't necessary to have relatives in Kansas City in order to be unhappy."

—GROUCHO MARX

Many people stay stuck because they are receiving big payoffs for staying the way that they are. Here are twenty-five common payoffs:

1. **No responsibility:** If you are sick, you don't have to take out the garbage, get a job, earn a living, get up in the morning and be somebody.
2. **Avoid suffering:** Somehow you view staying the way you are as a way to avoid the pain of life.
3. **Avoid rejection:** You could be choosing to stay overweight in order to avoid being rejected by members of the opposite sex. You can use your excess weight as an excuse to avoid dating.
4. **Get taken care of:** This is a biggie. As long as you stay sick, then other people have to make

your meals, do the chores around the house, or support you financially.

5. **Superiority:** You are so important and your issues are so special that no one can heal you. You might have to go to a specialist in another country, for God's sake, or find someone with multiple initials behind their name because you are so important even your problems can't be solved with ordinary solutions.

6. **No commitment:** You don't have to commit yourself to an exercise or eating plan. You can just do whatever you please.

7. **Permission:** Your illness or excess weight gives you permission to make excuses for yourself. You don't have to go to the party, wear a bathing suit, work long hours, or be accountable to other people.

8. **Sympathy:** Another biggie. Being sick or overweight may be the only way you know how to get attention.

9. **Freedom:** Being sick, you can finally quit your job and do whatever you want to do.

10. **Stay independent:** You don't have to listen to the experts. You can just keep doing whatever you want to do, eating whatever you like, and avoiding taking care of yourself because you would rather self-destruct than listen to anybody who actually knows how to make you better.

11. **Dependent on others:** You can keep other people at your beck and call because you can't do it yourself.

12. **Guilt:** You can use your illness or excess weight as a way to manipulate other people. They have to come and visit, stay married to you or neglect their own needs because you are so unwell.

13. **Control:** Your needs are so specific that you have to control everything about your environment. You decide what goes in the pantry, the lighting, the noise level, etc. It's all about what you need.

14. **Victim/Martyr:** Another biggie. You get attention by suffering. You are a victim of other people. You take on everybody's troubles and woes.

15. **No decisions:** You don't have to make choices because you are simply too tired to think straight.

16. **Apathy:** You can't possibly address the real issues in your life because you are too busy being sick or overweight.

17. **Attention:** Any type of attention, really. Even negative attention will do for you.

18. **Manipulation:** You use your condition to manipulate other people. You are so unwell their lives have to revolve around meeting your needs.

19. **Security:** Because you have an incurable whatever, other people, including even possibly the government's permanent disability program, have to take care of you for life.

20. **Blame:** You are so sick because someone else has hurt you. It's all the other person's fault. If

only this person hadn't been so horrible you could be living a normal life.

21. **Identity:** You are your illness. You are a card-carrying member of the incurable disease support group and your entire social life revolves around being a member of a sick group of people.

22. **Safety:** It's a lot easier to lie around the house being sick or overweight then it is to go out and take a risk in life.

23. **Avoidance of intimacy:** How could you possibly have sex or form a relationship when you feel so bad?

24. **Avoidance of listening:** You feel so bad, you just don't have the energy to listen to other people or care about their issues.

25. **Grow up:** Being sick keeps you in a permanent state of infancy. Other people make decisions for you, pay your bills, and make long-term plans on your behalf.

Getting better will change your life—and not just because you will get out of pain. You have to be ready on all levels to be a fully functioning human being, ready to be part of society, ready to be happy.

If I recognize that you are staying stuck in a payoff, I work with you to clear that. Sit with yourself and ask, at the end of the day, if your payoff is really worth it.

Chapter 54. Readiness

"Would you rather be right or free?"

—Byron Katie

Many times there is something that needs to take place before you will be ready to be healthy. That means you are putting things off. You don't need to use psychic gifts to tell if a person is waiting to be happy or healthy. All you really have to do is listen to his or her language. Statements that begin with, "I will be happy when..." are the best examples of this.

"I will be happy when the mortgage is paid off, the kids are out of college, my football team finally gets its act together, my boss quits, I get a better job, my spouse earns more money."

Or, "I can lose weight when there is not as much stress in my life."

Or, "I can get well after I retire and finally have time to exercise and take care of myself."

You get my drift. Do you have conversations like this? If there is something outside yourself that you are waiting for in order to get well, then you are waiting to be ready. If you notice you are waiting, then it is important to do the inner work or receive a healing to clear your conscious or subconscious blocks. Readiness means that you are ready to prosper on all levels right now, without waiting for anything.

To me, readiness is a spiritual attitude because life only happens right now. Now is all you have. If you wait to be healthy and happy, then you may never give yourself permission to allow the experience.

CHAPTER 55. ABLE

"The best path to happiness is learning to change as rapidly as life does."

—DON MIGUEL RUIZ

Once again, if you think you are not able to be healthy, you are putting the source that you need outside yourself. You think that you are not able to be well. The good news is that in the medical literature, almost every possible illness that you can think of has been healed.

If somebody else did it, then you can, too; you are actually able to heal, if you can just figure out how. Believing you are able to heal is essential. As long as you think you can't, you can't; if you think you can, you can. You believe there is something that you are missing. In all actuality, there is never a vacuum because vacuums don't actually exist in the universe.

God is amazingly abundant. When you realize that you always have everything you need to be happy and healthy right now, in this moment, all you have to do is open your eyes and discover your resources.

I worked with a lady in Kenya who had a serious illness. She did not have access to herbs and supplements, flower essences, or any of the usual holistic remedies that I commonly use. She didn't even have access to Western medicine, and her job took her out into the wilds of Africa for months at a time.

Listening to her story made me so thankful to work in the United States, where we have access to all kinds of healing remedies, both holistic and traditional. However, this dear woman was a big cat researcher. She and her husband had worked for decades to help preserve lions, tigers, and leopards all over the world.

We spoke about the tradition of shamanism, a practice of attaining altered states of consciousness in order to communicate with the spirit world. I taught her how to call on her power animals, which were the big cats, and ask them to facilitate her healing.

She understood completely and was deeply comforted. Where she had devoted her entire life to helping them, on a spiritual level they could now return the favor.

You always have everything you already need in order to get better. The first place to look is always to journey inward.

Chapter 56. Ready, Willing, and Able

"A Zen master's life is one continuous mistake."

—Dogen Zenji

Once you know that you are ready, willing, and able to heal, then the job is relatively easy, even if it takes you the next couple of years to be complete with your process. The next step is always to ask your mind, body, and soul, "What do I need now in order to get better?" In other words, what is your next step?

Personally, I am very good at steps. I have helped clients overcome the following challenges:

- Learning disabilities
- Head injuries
- Depression
- Anxiety
- Alcoholism
- Eating disorders
- Prostate cancer

- Hepatitis
- Shoulder pain
- Knee pain
- Hip pain
- Foot pain
- Neck pain
- Broken hands
- Weight problems
- Digestive disorders
- Parasites
- Chronic fatigue
- Fibromyalgia

Every journey is 1,000 steps. The key is to use the available power of your limitless intuition and figure out which step you are on and then take the next one. The key is to keep moving forward. Here are some possible questions to ask your guidance:

- What is my next step on the physical level?
- What is my next step energetically?
- What is my next step emotionally?
- What is my next step mentally?
- What is my next step spiritually?

By breaking things down into a series of small, comfortable steps, you make your process easier.

CHAPTER 57. MOVING FORWARD

"I'll go anywhere as long as it's forward."

—DAVID LIVINGSTONE

If you are exploring the interior of Africa trying to find the source of the Nile, keep moving. You may suffer from pneumonia, cholera, ulcers, and witness 400 people being massacred, but just keep going. That's what the great explorer David Livingstone did.

The thing about exploratory personal growth is that it's not actually a linear process. I have orchids in my studio where I work, and it is so fun to watch them grow. I have a chartreuse cattleya orchid, for example, that just surprises me. It may sit there for months with me watering it and looking at it. It seems like it's doing nothing. Then, all of a sudden, I will look over and there will be a new green shoot. Then that shoot will form what looks like a bud. Then the bud will divide into two and, all of a sudden, it seems to be moving in slow motion right before my eyes. The next thing you know there is the most beautiful orchid you have ever seen, chartreuse petals and a purple throat, reaching out to me and smiling like it's just saying hello and glad to be there.

People are that way also. It takes energy to heal. It takes time to process. You may think that nothing is happening inside you, and then, voila, you are ready for your next step.

So it is okay if on your life journey there are periods of rest and reflection, stepping back to assimilate the changes you have made. Maybe your next step is rest. Rest is a verb, and I am very big on encouraging other people to rest because while you are resting you *assimilate*. Assimilation is a very important process.

When you assimilate, you take in everything you have learned and you make it your own. Give yourself permission to honor your own growth process. It will be unique to you, and probably not exactly the way that other people do it. Even if hundreds of thousands of other people have overcome cancer or back pain or shoulder pain, the way you will do it— how, when, and why—will be your own way.

By staying in a process of constant discovery, always checking in with your intuition for guidance, you will be moving forward in a process of deep spiritual growth.

PART V:

ANGELS AND SPIRIT GUIDES

CHAPTER 58. GUIDES AND ANGELS

"I saw that there are many laws by which we are governed—spiritual laws, physical laws, and universal laws—most of which we have only an inkling. When we recognize these laws and learn how to use their positive and negative forces, we will have access to power beyond comprehension."

—BETTY J. EADIE

You have spiritual guides. Everybody has angels. You may call them your spiritual guides or you may call them your angels. Whatever you call them they are here for you. Even if you have never met them, they are with you here on your life journey.

They are with you every moment of every day of your life. I have usually about seventeen angels working with me. I like to joke that I need a lot of help to keep myself out of trouble!

People who work with others usually have more angels than those who work in solitary professions. These angels are located in your energy field. That means they literally surround you with their love and guidance, all the time, 24/7. You are never without them.

If you learn how, you can communicate with them, and rather easily. Of course, the first step is to be willing! Even with all my experience and practice, I am still surprised by how much love and guidance is constantly surrounding all of us. I think that one day, when we are all on the other side and have a chance to know how much we have been loved and guided during this lifetime, we will probably all have a totally different realization about our current experiences.

I like to teach people how to talk to their angels. This is one of the quickest and simplest ways to access your psychic gifts. When you start connecting to your angels you will know, hear, feel, and see much more information then you did before. This will make you better informed about what you need to know right now, for sure, but talking with your angels goes way beyond information. You will feel literally lifted up and comforted.

Once you learn how to talk to your angels, you will never feel alone in your life ever again. Even if you are completely by yourself in the middle of the woods or alone in your home, they are there with you, waiting to help you.

Your angels are like your team. They are part of the reason why you are never without resources and how you can always connect to the next step that will make you happier and healthier. That is a wonderful feeling: to know that you are always guided.

Chapter 59. Talking to Heaven

"You are not here to verify,
Instruct yourself, or inform curiosity
Or carry report. You are here to kneel
Where prayer has been valid. And prayer is more
Than an order of words, the conscious occupation
Of the praying mind, or the sound of the voice
praying."

—T.S. Eliot

I am going to teach you a rather simple way to talk to your guides and angels. The first step, as I said, is to be willing.

Sometimes people feel a little silly, or a little dubious. Search inside yourself and find out if there is anything that would prevent you from having this direct, spiritual connection.

On a mental level, it is helpful to recognize that even scientists recognize that only a very small portion of the known universe can be measured, analyzed, or proven. There is more to your life than meets the naked eye.

On a spiritual level, believe that you are already good enough to talk to your angels. No matter what mistakes you have made in your past, know that you are loved just the way you are.

Step One: Clear Your Energy

It is important to clear your energy. You will want to clear your energy because you don't want to experience any outside interference from having this direct spiritual connection.

I happened to grow up in the Christian tradition. I also respect all the world's religions and all the spiritual traditions. If these words below don't feel right to you, then I invite you to change the wording and use the words that resonate with your soul.

Rub your hands together. Rubbing your hands together generates chi. As you rub your hands together, imagine that you are gathering up any and all resistance to having a direct conversation with the divine. Then pass your hands over your head three times.

I like to say:

I CLEAR MY ENERGY IN THE NAME OF
GOD THE FATHER.

I CLEAR MY ENERGY IN THE NAME OF
JESUS THE SON.

I CLEAR MY ENERGY IN THE NAME OF
THE HOLY GHOST.

When I do my clearing, I usually feel a tingling. It's sort of the feeling you get when you know your room needs to be vacuumed. It's about time you cleared your energy field, and you know it. Keep clearing your energy field until you feel completely neutral.

How do you know when your energy field is clear? You will feel calm on the inside. If you shut your eyes and look, your energy field will look smooth. You will feel centered. You will feel free of any outside interference.

Step Two: Calibrate a Yes and a No

This should be easy, so start by making it easy for yourself by getting a clear yes and no. I recommend you do this every time in case your energy is not as settled as you think it is.

Stand up and relax your whole body. Breathe. Breathe into all five corners of yourself. Breathe into your legs and feet. Breathe into your arms and your hands. Breathe up into your head. Feel the chi radiating throughout your whole body. Then, shut your eyes.

Say to yourself, ANGEL SPIRIT GUIDES, SHOW ME A YES.

Then, keeping your eyes shut, watch inside yourself for what happens.

More than likely you may sway just slightly forward. You will feel a gentle shift in your weight, as if you are slightly leaning forward.

However, the reason I am encouraging you to calibrate your yes and your no is that some of you may sway to the right or the left. It really doesn't matter. Just find out how your angels want to communicate with you.

Now, if you are not getting a clear signal, that is a sign that your energy is really not actually clear. I encourage you to go back and repeat step one. Clear your energy again. It's okay. It really means that you have some resistance. You are normal. Most of your conversations happen with other humans and maybe sometimes your pets.

Once you have a clear yes, then also ask for a clear no. Say, ANGEL SPIRIT GUIDES, PLEASE SHOW ME A CLEAR NO. More than likely, your weight will shift backward or in the reverse direction as the yes.

The angels really actually want to communicate with you. They are always rooting for you all the time. They want to make this easy for you. If you are still having trouble, say out loud, ANGEL SPIRIT GUIDES, PLEASE MAKE THIS SUPER EASY FOR ME. And they will.

Step Three: Ask Permission

Your angels and spiritual guides are here to protect you, to guide you, to help you with everything you are here to accomplish during your time here on Earth. That means they are here for you, not for anybody else. Therefore, when you talk to them, don't ask for other people, ask for yourself.

For example, if you ask, "Angel spirit guides,

do I have permissions to ask questions about my neighbors' sex life?" You will more than likely get a clear no—as in a hell no. That is none of your business.

You can start by asking, "Angel spirit guides, do I have permission at this time to talk about _____?" And here you would include the subject matter that you want to ask about. Timing is everything. Sometimes your angels don't mind talking to you about something, but it's just not the right time.

If you have ever been in a relationship of any kind, you know what I am talking about. There is something that is bothering you but it's just not the right time to deal with it. There are other more important issues that you had better be looking at first. Start by talking with your angels about what is most important right now.

Step Four: Highest Best Interests

When I am working with my clients, I like to joke about this. Don't ask questions like, "Can I eat a hot fudge sundae?" or "Can I lie down in the middle of the road?" These are what I call stupid questions.

The answer to the above would be yes, of course, you can do that. You could eat a hot fudge sundae, and you could lie down in the middle of the interstate.

A smarter question would be, "Is it in my highest best interest to eat a hot fudge sundae at this time?" Your answer could be totally different! Or, perhaps, "Is it in my highest best interest to lie down in the middle of the road at this time?" Hopefully not!

I like to ask highest best interest questions because these are also highest good questions.

When you ask in your highest best interest, believe it or not, the answer will be in the highest good of all. Because you are part of the whole, and God is all there is, then it's all God and, therefore, it's all good. You can't make a choice that is in your highest best interest that is also, at the end of the day, not also good for everyone you know and even the whole world.

Because everything that happens is subtly dependent on everything else, when you make a choice in your life that moves you toward your own highest best interest, then you are actually moving forward, spiritually speaking, and you are subtly helping other people move forward, even if it is only by your example.

When you make a choice that is in your highest best interest, you are raising your personal vibration, and that benefits everybody on the planet.

Step Five: Ask and You Shall Receive

Once you are clear on the other four steps, you are now ready to ask your questions. Standing up in the middle of your room, ask highest best interest questions. I like to keep things in simple yes or no questions with all my clients starting out.

Years ago, I helped a woman with special needs lose forty-five pounds. I broke everything down into small easy steps. After that, I thought, I need to keep things simple for everybody. Simple is the way!

Often in life, the simplest answer is the one that you

will have the easiest time implementing. Philosophy refers to this as Occam's Razor. Other issues being equal, a simpler way is more often superior to a more complex one. If I gave you 535 things to do, more than likely, you are going to get so overwhelmed you may not be able to accomplish even one of them. So when you keep things simple for yourself, asking highest best interest questions, you can find your next steps rather easily.

You can ask, "Is it in my highest best interest to take my next step on the physical level, the energetic level, the emotional level, the mental level, or the spiritual level?" Once you know which level you need to work on next, you can narrow it down further. For example, if you get that it is in your highest best interest to work on the physical level, you can ask, "Is it in my highest best interests today to take a walk, see a chiropractor, or go to the health food store?"

Sometimes maybe there are fifteen things you could do to be healthier, but perhaps one or two of those are absolutely critical and will take you the farthest toward a significant change.

CHAPTER 60. THE BRAIN LIKES THINGS IN BITS AND PIECES

"I believe in intuitions and inspirations...I sometimes FEEL that I am right. I do not KNOW that I am."

—ALBERT EINSTEIN

You have a part of your brain called the amygdala. The amygdala is the "fight, flight, or freeze" part of your brain, and is considered part of the limbic system. You actually have two amygdalae on either side, located inside your head at the level of your eyes. When information comes into your brain, your amygdala takes control of it and says, "I am going to think logically about this, stay calm, and handle it," or, "OMG, what is going on? This is really scary; I can't handle it!"

When the amygdala does not recognize the information as a threat, the information gets sent to the higher reasoning aspects of your brain. When the amygdala recognizes the incoming energy as a threat, then the signals get sent to the back of your brain, your reptilian reflexes, where you just react out of old programming. If you are reacting, you are acting like your dumb old self—you know the one, the person you were before you knew any better.

One of the ways to make the smartest changes in life is to make change so small, easy, and unthreatening that your amygdala does not freak out and go into overload. Even if you say you want to be healthy, if you are willing, ready, and able to be radiantly healthy, if I were to say to you, "Okay, we are going to radically change your life. A year from now you are going to be juicing, exercising every day, dealing with your issues, getting back in touch with your spiritual self, and staying on a regular program of healthy eating," your amygdala could potentially shut the whole thing down and leave you sprinting off in the other direction.

Gentle is the way. I am a gentle person and I like to work gently. Humor is the way. Even though I am not a comedian, I like to have a sense of humor about things, because humor also bypasses the amygdala.

At the end of the day, life itself is a sexually induced situation that is going to end up for all of us in the cold locker. Not a single one of us is going to get out of here alive. We are all just spiritual beings having a human experience, and not one of us meets any scientific description of perfect. Not even close. Just ask your family back home—the one your child self grew up with—and they will probably be more than happy to tell you everything they think is wrong with you.

And yet what you are going through now, whatever it is, no matter how much you are suffering right now, is exactly where you need to be. So the key is to be super easy on yourself. Love is the way. When you are loving and kind to yourself and keep things easy, you can find your next steps.

CHAPTER 61. CHANNELING ANGELS

"If you exist in a feeling of love—if you can find it in everything you do, transmit it through your touch, through your words, eyes and feelings—you can cancel out with one act of love thousands of acts of a lower nature."

—SANAYA ROMAN

Once you get good at asking simple yes and no questions, then you can begin having deeper, more complex conversations with your angels. I have found that keeping a journal of my interactions with angels helps me to make sense of the messages I receive.

I have been writing journals for well over thirty-six years. My journals have allowed me to keep in close contact with my soul and how I really feel. Over the years, I have recorded my triumphs and my sorrows, what I ate five times a day, how I exercised, and what my angels have advised me.

You, too, can keep a journal of not only your

ordinary life events but also what your angel guides are talking to you about. Now, as important as this information is, I want to start by saying that it is important also not to hold onto old energy. Releasing old energy helps to clear the things from our life that can delay our spiritual growth.

Several years ago, I noticed that my journals were taking over my house. I had journals literally stretching back to when I was seventeen years old. I asked a friend to help me burn my old journals. I was having trouble finding where to store my new ones, as so many of the records I had carefully kept on acid-free paper were jamming up every possible cabinet, shelf, the wine cellar, under the bed and in my drawers. It was absolutely ridiculous. I asked my friend to help me, and he began by putting a log on the fire in my fireplace. Big mistake! He had no idea how many journals I actually had.

We started burning my journals about seven o'clock one evening and ended well after one a.m. We burned so many journals that the wood on the floor next to the fireplace got scorched.

I was lucky that night that I didn't actually burn down my house, but I reckoned that my angels, once again, were taking care of me. I am starting by advising you to channel your angels, but not to hold onto your records for too long.

How long is too long? You can ask. For me, it is usually about a year. But sometimes you know intuitively that you are going through a major passage in your life and that you will need to hold onto your messages from your angels longer than that, so that you can keep going and keep re-reading their encouragement.

I recently went through a two-and-a-half–year period of intense change.

I kept my journals throughout that time, and they helped me keep moving forward; I would go back and reread what my angels said to me at the beginning of my changes. It was like rereading my pep talks. But maybe a good rule of thumb is to start each January by letting go of the old energy.

The change in me after letting go of my old journals—the ones I had kept since I was seventeen— that long night by the fire was surprisingly huge. I let go of layers and layers and layers of old energy. Every time I sat by the fire and read something from those years past, it touched my heart. It was all very sweet. But it was important to let go of the old energy in order to be fully in the present.

I am just like everybody else, i.e., human, and I get busy and interested in many other activities, so I forget to take time to talk to my angels and listen to what they have to say. Then I go through days of being woken up in the middle of the night and I remember to get back on track.

You can set aside time to talk to your angels. Find a quiet time of the day, whether it is first thing in the morning, late at night before bed, or during a rest period of your working day. By using the simple skills I have taught you about getting yes or no answers from angels, and recording the answers in a journal, you can gain better understanding of the messages that are available to you.

Chapter 62. List Your Angels

> "The Ascended Masters, together with the angels and Archangels, teach us how to liberate ourselves and others."
>
> —Elizabeth Clare Prophet

Everybody has a primary guardian angel, but more than likely, you have other angels also. Take out a pen and piece of paper. Get very quiet by yourself in a place you know you won't be disturbed. Say a prayer of thanksgiving and ask your angels to reveal themselves to you.

Here is a prayer I suggest, but I also recommend speaking directly and frankly from your own heart if that would feel more comfortable for you.

Angel Spirit Guides,
Thank you so much for guiding and protecting
me all the days of my life. I love you. Thank you
for loving me and helping me on my way.

Thank you for all you do to guide me in my spiritual growth. I would like to know you better. Please show your faces to me. Please tell me your names. Please help me understand what you are all about. I love you. I appreciate you. I thank you from the bottom of my heart. Amen.

I used to keep a list of my angels and their functions in my old journals but, of course, that first list has long since been burned in my fireplace. I just ask again, and I know with whom I am working.

More than likely, you will have angels who are good at what you do. For example, I have several angels who are good at healing. It makes me laugh, but I have an angel who is a cook, not a chef. And that's how I am—I don't view myself as any kind of gourmet cuisine expert—it's just a "Let's get this dinner done" type of thing.

I have an angel who is good at beading, and beading is my hobby. I have an angel who is an herbalist.

And I absolutely adore my power animals. My primary power animal is a mother snow leopard. She is magnificent. She doesn't talk a lot, and when she does, she keeps it short and sweet. She is the spiritual guide who allows me to guide people to make major leaps in their lives. She has helped me leap out of many messes in my own life with grace and ease. I have often seen myself riding on her back as she helps me take yet another giant leap forward.

I also have a baby snow leopard, who is all about fun. She always wants to keep playing, no matter what I am doing. She has a sense of humor and is warm and cuddly and funny.

I have a hawk, who allows me to keep an eye on the big picture. Whenever I am going for a walk and see a hawk, I remind myself to speak to my hawk and ask for a view of the world. I can telescope my vision and see bigger and bigger and bigger, thanks to my hawk.

And lastly, I work with a hummingbird. Hummingbirds are tiny but full of endless joy. Hummingbird reminds me to find the ecstasy in even the smallest moments, lying in my hammock on my porch staring up at the sky, giving my dog Belle a bath, teaching my little yoga class, walking through my herb garden. The hummingbird is all about quiet, unheralded moments of complete ecstasy.

To get to know your angels and spiritual guides, quiet yourself and ask them to tell you more about who they are, what they are good at, and what they are here to help you with. They may reveal themselves to you in all kinds of funny ways.

You could see them in your mind's eye, or hear their distinctive voices. You could feel their presence around you, or simply know that you are not alone.

I keep a list of my angels at the back of my current journal so that when I want specific help on a particular subject, I can figure out which ones I want to talk to.

Just like you probably keep the number of your accountant handy, and know to call him or her when you have a tax question, by keeping a list of your angels, you will know whom to call about specific subjects.

Chapter 63. Getting Quiet

"Notice what your mind is actually doing now. You don't have to seek to do this. You're already fully equipped. You don't have to go anywhere or do anything special. Simply make just seeing your intention. That's all."

—Steve Hagen

When you channel your angels, it's all about listening. This is where meditation comes in. When you have practiced quieting your mind, you will become better at knowing when your guides are really trying to get your attention.

You can start in the middle of the night—not that I am an advocate of interrupting your sleep, but often this is the time of day when there is the least interference. The rest of your family will be asleep, even your dogs and cats, most likely.

I know sometimes my sleep gets interrupted and I can't go back to sleep until I write down whatever it is that my angels want to say to me. If your partner doesn't mind, go in the next room and pull out your journal and a pen. Clear your energy. Figure out which angel wants to speak to you. More than likely, they each have different voices and different ways of speaking.

I hear from my guardian angel frequently during the day. He looks like a rock star. He seems to have male energy, with long, flowing, curly, brown hair, and he sometimes seems to be carrying a white board upon which is written major messages for me. "Don't worry, we have got your back. All will be well!" he says.

You would think sometimes if you talk to your angels that you will get these profound messages, and frequently they are, but don't be surprised if you hear, "Have a nice day!" "Remember to have fun!" or "Be at peace."

My snow leopard mother, as I have mentioned, speaks in short sentences. Often she is just sleeping. If I see her in my mind's eye and she is poised for a leap, then I know something major is happening. She has a kindness and gentleness about her, but recently I saw her bare her teeth. It wasn't a threatening gesture, in the least. It was more like, "We are on a roll here, and I have got your back."

Once you know who is speaking to you, just start writing. Write down as fast as you can so that there is no left brain interference. Don't stop to interrupt yourself to reread what it is they are saying to you. You can do that later, in the morning, or when the messages seem to have come to a complete stop.

Sometimes I go back and reread even months later what my angels have said to me, and I am still amazed. Often they give me advance warning, or they tell me what I am supposed to do. It could be a paragraph that you write, or it could be a few pages.

Your angels may show you pictures in your mind's eye. This would be accessing your gift of psychic vision. Or you could also feel certain feelings. Allow the communication that comes to open all the gifts so that you receive what you need to know in stereo learning.

You will know when your angels are done because you will feel like you are finally able to go back to sleep. Or they will simply stop speaking and the communication will come to a halt. As I mentioned, it's often easiest to channel in the middle of the night because of the deep quiet we find in the night. But as you get better at this, you can channel your angels any time of day.

If you practice writing down what you hear, then when you hear their voices other times of the day, you will know who it is that you are actually hearing from.

As I have taught numerous clients how to communicate with their angels over the years, I have occasionally had to do a healing to clear the blocks to a person being willing to enter into divine dialogue.

Even though the techniques I teach are relatively simple and easy, it is our own emotional blocks that often keep us from receiving the guidance that our souls crave.

The first step is to know that you are loved unconditionally, just the way you are right now. The second step is to know that you are always guided, every moment of every day of your life. There is never a second that you are not totally taken care of; it's just up to you to pay attention and listen. The third step is to know that you don't have to do anything to deserve this divine guidance. You are already worthy, you are already good enough. No matter what mistakes you feel you have made in the past, your angels are always there waiting to guide you.

I think many of us have never experienced this level of love and support. Most of what we have experienced in the way of support has been conditional, spotty, there and then not there. People may let you down, break your heart, and disappoint you, but your angels will never, ever let you down. Learning how to embrace this level of love and support can radically change our experience of life if we allow the guidance to flow through to us.

Chapter 64. What to Avoid

"Intuition functions in a quantum leap. It has no methodological procedure, it simply sees things."

—Osho

I like to teach people of all ages, shapes, and sizes how to talk to their angels and how to get their own guidance, but there are some kinds of people that I like to work with more before going on to this level. If a person is on any kind of psychiatric medication, that is a pretty good indication that he or she is having trouble dealing with what is known as ordinary reality.

This is not a judgment of any kind. Everybody is always doing the best they can, choosing what they know to be their good with the knowledge they have at the moment. And I know that is true.

I don't think that doctors or psychiatrists or psychologists are evil or bad. I actually think they have a very hard job. But what I know to be true is that psychiatric drugs and what I call "stupid drugs," i.e. marijuana, cocaine, and other psychedelic equivalents, all clog up your energy field and interfere with the energetic connection to the divine. To get clear guidance, you will need to be clear. And you can't be clear when you are taking any drug that is interfering with your mind.

If you are taking any medication that is affecting you mentally, talk to your doctor and work through your issues to get clearer before taking the steps I am talking about.

Years ago, I taught a class about healing the chakras. I taught everybody in the class how to draw a picture of their own aura. Nobody thought they could do it. Nobody thought they could even see their aura, but everybody in the class could, and more easily than they had previously realized.

One man in the class had taken what I call "stupid drugs" years ago. When he drew his aura, he could literally see the energetic residue of the stupid drugs as a red cloud above his head. When you interfere with your spiritual connection, you create the potential for some of the deepest depressions of all.

On the positive side, when we keep our energy field clear, when we maintain this deep spiritual connection and spiritual communication going, we feel not only guided and protected, we are able to access our own inner strength and power, and that gives us a sense of deep inner happiness that nobody can take away.

After the gentleman saw for himself what was in his aura, which happened maybe twenty years before and when he was less aware, I did a healing with him to clear his field so that he could access his divine connection.

It is not uncommon for negative spiritual energies to reside in this kind of energetic debris. I had to clear the negative spiritual energies that had been with him for a long time.

I remember once being with a woman who had been on psychiatric medication for about thirty years. It was like her energy field was full of static. If you are old enough to remember the old-time TV sets, the kind where if you switched stations there was a black and white static field, that is what her entire energy field felt like. It was like she was constantly switching on and switching off, unable to maintain a clear spiritual connection. I felt a deep compassion for her; she had also been suffering mightily for many years and did not know how to make herself better.

Now, I am not advocating rushing out and flushing your drugs down the toilet. A better approach is, if you are on any form of medication that affects your mental/emotional field, to learn how to heal your brain naturally. This is much easier than you realize.

If you figure out what your brain chemistry is missing, you can start rather easily by giving yourself the amino acids and other nutrients you need in order to start getting better. Amino acids are the building blocks of protein, so it is important, if you are having or have had some kind of brain problem, that you include enough high-quality protein in your diet.

It takes courage to face and clear your emotional and mental issues. Once again, I like to look for the root causes, deal with the root issues, and then medication no longer becomes a necessity. I have helped more people get off psychiatric drugs than I can even count.

You have to be willing to find a better way, you have to decide you want to be done with the old ways of inadequate coping, and then you can move forward. But, if you are serious about developing your intuitive abilities, realize that you may be very gifted, intuitively speaking, but that as long as you are on "stupid drugs" or even medically prescribed psychiatric drugs, you will not be able to get or maintain a totally clear connection.

If I have a client who wants to develop his or her intuition and is on these drugs, I generally encourage them to do their deeper healing before developing this other aspect of themselves.

A woman who once came to me wanted me to train her how to be a medical intuitive. She told me that people ask her all the time what is wrong with them and that she is usually right. However, she was on antidepressants, she wasn't able to make a living as a realtor, and she thought she would just pick up a side business helping people with their health. As they say, physician, heal thyself.

Although none of us is perfect, and we are all on our journey, if you are unwell in your own mind, it is a very good idea to start with yourself. Realize that you are part of the whole.

If you don't think you are worth healing, then deep down you won't believe that other people are either. You can only take other people as far as you have gone yourself. There is a difference between knowing about something and actually holding and embodying the energy yourself. Who you are speaks louder than anything you can say or do.

I have healed so many things in myself I have almost gotten to the point where I said, "Okay, God, I promise, I will read about it in a book! I can research this. I don't need to have every illness on the planet in order to learn how to be a healer. Thank you for sharing."

Chapter 65. Healing Yourself May Take a Surprise

"Be at peace and see a clear pattern and plan running through all your lives, nothing is by chance."

—Eileen Caddy

As we learn how to navigate the trap doors in our own mind, we begin to develop compassion for other people and how hard it is for so many to face themselves and actually get better.

A client of mine once lamented the fact that nobody else in her family was doing any kind of spiritual growth work. They all ate junk food, took drugs, drank diet sodas, and weren't all that spiritually aware. I asked her how many years she had been working on herself. At that point, it had been maybe ten or twelve years. I asked her how much money she had spent on her own growth work. She couldn't even count.

It often takes special circumstances for people to be able to take the first step. Sometimes things have to become so challenging that people give up and say, "Okay, help me!" Newton's first law of physics states that an object at rest remains at rest and an object in motion stays in motion with the same speed and in the same direction unless acted upon by an unbalanced force. What does an unbalanced force look like in an ordinary life?

An unbalanced force could be a sudden diagnosis. It could be losing your job. It could be your spouse asking for a divorce, your child leaving the home, the death of your parents, pet, or a close friend. It could be a robbery, your roof leaking, a car wreck, or your house burning down.

You can read all the self-help or diet books in the world but not take the first step. What it takes for you to heal yourself may actually be something totally unexpected that moves you inexorably into a new direction. You may need a surprise visit from the divine disguised as a breakdown.

PART VI:

DEALING WITH PAIN

Chapter 66. The Blessing of The Breakdown

"Concerning all acts of initiative (and creation), there is one elementary truth, the ignorance of which kills countless ideas and splendid plans; that the moment one definitely commits oneself, then Providence moves too."

—Johann Wolfgang von Goethe

Once a dear friend of mine asked me about her brother. He was a severe alcoholic and had ended up in the I.C.U. with liver failure. He actually broke out of the I.C.U. to go get himself another drink. Another time, he was committed to a mental hospital and then broke out in the middle of the night to go get another drink. He could just not be stopped.

Even though you would think that he might have suffered enough already, he had not yet received the blessing of a breakdown. My friend asked me if there was anything at all she could do to help her brother.

I get this question all the time in different ways from other people. What about my sister, father, brother, mother, husband, wife, child, aunt, cousin?

Maybe they have not yet received the blessing of a breakdown. It is easy for people just to keep going on their path, no matter how dysfunctional, uncomfortable, or insane it is. Sometimes the thought of change is scarier than the thought of just keeping on with what you know. Sometimes God has to step in.

You know for sure when God has stepped in when you are suddenly facing a challenge not of your own choosing. "Now THIS?" you may ask indignantly. "I went through all this stuff already, and now you are giving me THIS?" Allow yourself to have a moment, an hour, a day of pity partying and then get on with it. As they say, sometimes when your foundations are shaking, maybe God is the one doing the shaking.

It all goes back to chaos theory. In order to shift to a higher vibration, you have to go into chaos. In fact, the greater the mess you feel like you are in, congratulations! Although nobody likes to suffer, and it is not fun to receive a diagnosis you weren't expecting, I still say, "Congratulations! You have received the blessing of a breakdown!" If you take that attitude, then all will be well. Love yourself enough to get better. Then you will really know what it actually takes to help other people get better.

About two years ago, I injured my right shoulder. The first thing I thought when it happened was, "It's obviously my turn." The irony was that I had helped countless other people heal their own shoulders.

Now, shoulders are fairly complicated, as there are eleven different movements of the shoulder joint and lots of layers of little muscles, any one of which can throw the whole thing out of balance. I had studied the shoulders inside and out, little realizing that one day I would need that information for myself.

As per the usual, I went through all the layers. Was it physical? Yes. Was it energetic? Yes. Was it emotional? Yes. Was it mental? Yes. I knew I could get better, but there was definitely a thought pattern I had been holding onto that affected my shoulder. Was it spiritual? Yes! I was being guided in another direction and needed to hurt my shoulder in order to find my way there. The root cause was a weakness in my heart after a particularly sharp emotional pain.

That weakness in my heart on an energetic and emotional level had translated over into weakness in the subscapularis muscle, the muscle underneath the shoulder blade, which eventually threw my entire right shoulder out of balance. It was actually a freak accident that injured it. I was reviewing a class on healing work for the muscles and had poor body mechanics while trying to help a gentleman with very tight legs. Then a few months later I felt the tendons and ligaments rip while teaching yoga, and then I reinjured my shoulder for a third time while wielding a pickaxe in my garden.

After the third time, I decided I was really tired of hurting my shoulder and was determined to be complete with that particular lesson. Even though I had helped many other people with their shoulders, I had to learn the lesson in my own body. I hurt so badly it was difficult to lift my purse or take Belle for a walk. I had a hard time carrying anything, and the entire experience led me to re-evaluate how I was teaching yoga. I could not do a single down dog or whole body pushup. I had to think again and live my life differently from many perspectives. This is the blessing of the breakdown.

So when you fall and hit your head, get the lab report back, find out your spouse is leaving you, discover that all your money is actually gone, stop and ask yourself, "What is the blessing in this breakdown?"

Realize that you are actually receiving a blessing, and you can begin to transform the energy behind any diagnosis, behind any accident, behind any piece of apparently bad news.

CHAPTER 67. KNOW THE SPIRITUAL MESSAGE

"Be still, and know that I am God."

—PSALMS 46:9

I like to say that if I am in physics class, it is kind of helpful to know that I am supposed to be learning physics. If you are going through a particular challenge in your life, on the surface it may be about learning how to have a healthy relationship with food or how to heal your shoulder. But trust me, the lesson—the real lesson—will be much deeper than that.

If you go into a difficulty, you can figure out what it is that you are supposed to be learning, so that you can get the message and be done with the challenge. You won't need to be repeating yourself over and over again, because you've got it.

I always joke that it is more interesting to go on and face new challenges. In fact, you will know when you are actually growing when you are not facing the same challenges over and over again. If you find yourself facing the same lesson, you know you are not actually learning it.

Once I helped a lady recover who had suffered from diarrhea for over fifteen years. She had been everywhere, medically speaking, and had even begun studying shamanism as a means of learning self-healing. She had plenty of money so no resource was left unexamined. Finally, she came to me.

She had parasites. To me, this issue is so obvious, and yet many practitioners of all kinds never check for parasites. I explained to my client that parasites are all about you allowing someone else to eat your lunch. Deep down, it will mean that you have a "you lose, they win" paradigm going on inside. And it means, at least energetically, that you are codependent.

After I explained this pattern to her, she said, "Oh, my God. It's like I have swept that floor a hundred times already!" She had stopped drinking over seven years ago. I told her to give herself 500 points just for not being an alcoholic anymore. But the core energetic issue was still there.

The energetic pattern of "she loses, other people win," was deeply embedded in her energy field. No doctor or shaman had been able to shift that pattern before. We worked together to take her healing to a whole new level. She understood what her lesson was, but had not actually cleared it.

CHAPTER 68. THE FIRST STEP IS TO UNDERSTAND YOUR LESSON

"Love creates healing."

—SANAYA ROMAN

At the end of the day, the lesson behind any illness or challenge in your life will be spiritual. That is because you are a spiritual being having a human experience. You are just here to play, actually—at least that is my belief. You get to play with other humans who themselves are all practicing being a human. You may like how they are acting, you may not like how they are acting, but we are all just practicing.

Understanding your core spiritual lesson may go a long way to catapulting you out of any challenge in your life. Once you understand that your entire life is set up as a self-guided, self-directed, spiritual, self-study course, you can figure out whether you are in physics class, love yourself class, love others class, realize it is all good class, or what.

Maybe we are all just humans with faults who make errors of judgment, but it's all good because it's all part of our spiritual experience, and that there is nothing really to be afraid of, not now or ever. One of the biggest spiritual errors is to make the mistake of thinking that other people can do better than they are already currently doing. Another major error is to think that there is a measurable, objectifiable reality out there. In actuality, there is no *out there* out there. It's all just your projection. It's your inward journey projected outward. It's all your dream.

So when you are doing an intuitive reading of someone else, you are watching what the other person is dreaming and how their projection of that inward experience is playing out on the material level. Your physical body is actually the most dense, obvious expression of what you are habitually thinking, feeling, and experiencing.

When you want everything to be able to be weighed, measured, quantified, added up, lab tested, scientifically proven, and generally accepted as universally recognized theory, then you actually have a block to seeing the world as it is in this moment right now. Even astrophysicists will tell you that the known, measurable universe—you me, all the stars, and planets—makes up only *4 percent* of reality! That is why I started the earlier part of this book talking about the importance of love. Love yourself. Love other people. Love what you are doing. Love your life.

One of the most important affirmations you can ever make is, I LOVE MY LIFE. Love your life and all the characters in it. As you examine your own drama, you will find it has meaning, and even the so-called bad guys and the bit players have something important to offer you.

The higher your level of consciousness, the more you are aware of. And, the more you are aware of, the more other people start calling you intuitive, psychic, and in tune. Remember what I said earlier in the book: intuition is a byproduct of unconditional love. So when you really want to develop your intuitive gifts, get serious about your own spiritual growth, open your heart, and learn how you can be more loving.

For most of us, unconditional love is an attainable goal and is what most of traditional religion is here to teach us about, if we digest the actual messages:

"Love thy neighbor as thyself."

—THE BIBLE

"Honor thy father and thy mother."

—THE BIBLE

"Judge not lest you be judged."

—THE BIBLE

"The power of God is with you at all times; through the activities of mind, senses, breathing, and emotions; and is constantly doing all the work using you as a mere instrument."

—The Bhagavad-Gita

"No one who does good work will ever come to a bad end, either here or in the world to come"

—The Bhagavad-Gita

"The peace of God is with them whose mind and soul are in harmony, who are free from desire and wrath, who know their own soul."

—The Bhagavad-Gita

"He who sees me in all things, and all things in me, is never far from me, and I am never far from him."

—The Bhagavad-Gita

"Whatever you do, make it an offering to me -- the food you eat, the sacrifices you make, the help you give, even your suffering."

—The Bhagavad-Gita

"Still your mind in me, still yourself in me, and without a doubt you shall be united with me, Lord of Love, dwelling in your heart."

—The Bhagavad-Gita

3:31 Say: "If ye do love [hubb] Allah, follow me: Allah will love [ihbbikum] you and forgive you your sins: For Allah is Oft-Forgiving, Most Merciful."

—The Qur'an

"As human beings we all want to be happy and free from misery... we have learned that the key to happiness is inner peace. The greatest obstacles to inner peace are disturbing emotions such as anger, attachment, fear and suspicion, while love and compassion and a sense of universal responsibility are the sources of peace and happiness."

—Dalai Lama

"Where there is FAITH, there is LOVE; Where there is LOVE; there is PEACE; Where there is PEACE; there is GOD; Where there is GOD; there is BLISS."

—Sri Sathya Sai Baba

"The way is not in the sky. The way is in the heart."

—Buddha

"You, yourself, as much as anybody in the entire universe, deserve your love and affection."

—Buddha

"True unconditional love expects nothing in return"

—Dalai Lama

"If you want others to be happy, practice compassion.
"If you want to be happy, practice compassion."

—Dalai Lama

"Love will immediately enter into any mind that truly wants it."

—A Course in Miracles

"The search for love is but the honest searching out of everything that interferes with love."

—A Course in Miracles

"Your task is not to seek for love, but merely to seek and find all the barriers within yourself that you have built against it."

—A Course in Miracles

I am sure you have heard many if not all of these lessons before. Maybe now they will take on a new importance.

Chapter 69. Major Blocks to Spiritual Progress

"When you judge another, you do not define them, you define yourself."

—Wayne Dyer

It is true that there are many activities that accelerate our spiritual growth. I am a big fan of meditating and praying, for example. However, you can meditate for twenty years and still not get anywhere, spiritually speaking. In my mind, your spiritual lessons are actually going to be found in the most mundane aspects of your life:

- How you treat your children
- Whether or not you have overcome your distaste for exercise or healthy movement
- How you handle your emotions
- The choices you make, big and small, in everyday life

It's the little stuff—and how that little stuff shows up in your body as illness and diseases—that I think makes all the difference. It is my experience that to overcome any serious illness, at the end of the day, that in and of itself is what leads us to deep spiritual growth. You can't really stay your old bad self and get truly well.

Years ago, I worked with a man who was an accomplished amateur senior golfer. He doubted everything I did with him until he went out on the golf course and started beating everybody. Now that was fun! He asked me once if I thought it was trivial to work on being a better golfer. I told him no. "To be great at anything, you have to face yourself," I said.

You can pick up any thread in your life—aiming to be a better golfer, trying to overcome cancer, learning how to overcome an eating disorder, how to exercise without injuring yourself—and to get to the very end you will have to face very important lessons about yourself.

In my mind, these lessons are more important for your spiritual growth and more effective for actually moving you forward than all the rituals you do without thinking. Once again, it is true that spiritual people tend to meditate and pray, give money to charities, demonstrate kindness to others, or attend church or some other religious institution. Those activities will go a long way to improving your health and happiness.

But when we start looking at the major and minor bumps in the road from that bigger picture, from the hawk's eye view, it's not just cancer, it's your opportunity to seize the moment and for your soul to grow just as it is yearning to grow. It's not just your sore throat that's bothering you; it's your soul calling out for you to express yourself. You didn't just rip the tendons and ligaments in your shoulder. Maybe you weren't listening before that to a very important message from your heart.

A couple of years ago, I sat down with a new client who had prostate cancer. I told him he needed to stop feeling guilty. Guilt and shame weigh down the soul like nothing else. It's like trying to walk around with big rocks in your pockets. You just feel like you can never get anywhere.

This very accomplished gentleman had had a number of affairs. He wasn't getting what he needed in his marriage. "You are basically a very healthy guy," I told him. "Healthy guys have a sex drive. In fact, if I have a man and he has low sex drive, that is card-carrying proof that he is not healthy."

He wept. No one had ever spoken to him frankly and kindly about that. We worked together so that he could forgive himself. Healing the cancer was easy after that. I told him to spend four months with me. He was worried that conventional treatments for prostate cancer would not only be expensive, but could potentially also leave him impotent. I said that after four months, he should find the most obsessively detailed surgeon he could find to do multiple biopsies. After four months, he had those multiple biopsies and his cancer was, in fact, completely gone.

He had forgiven himself. He got the lesson. He not

only understood the lesson, he learned it and then he let it go. He didn't need the messenger any longer because he got the message.

CHAPTER 70. IT'S THE LITTLE THINGS THAT COUNT

"It has long been an axiom of mine that the little things are infinitely the most important."

—ARTHUR CONAN DOYLE

When you see the process of wellness as a process of deep spiritual growth, then you can start looking for all the gifts. After a long-term path of studying and practicing holistic healing, I enjoyed many years of radiant physical and emotional health. Then, one December, I got pneumonia.

Now, I am rarely if ever sick, so I was sort of in denial about the fact that I actually had pneumonia. I thought that I was going to get over pneumonia rather quickly. I thought I was going to turn the corner and wake up the next morning breathing normally; yet the thing kept going.

I was ramping up my chicken soup and herbs and

juicing. I was resting. I was doing everything that I could think of, and still thinking that tomorrow morning it would all be gone. It was the sickest I had been in over eighteen years, in fact.

After about a month, people started talking to me about antibiotics. I don't have anything against antibiotics, doctors, or traditional medicine—I believe that all treatments have their place and time—but I just usually choose door number 2, which is another way.

After a month, door number 2 was still not working, but I intuitively knew that my pneumonia was bigger than something that mere antibiotics could actually cure. I was facing a deep level of grief that was affecting my lungs. I hadn't even recognized that the grief was there. It took a major illness for me to see that. I was gentle with myself and this realization.

I remember a snow that came the next month, in February, after the pneumonia had finally gone. It rarely snows in Atlanta. I got up early that morning and went down to take pictures of the orchids with my iPhone, the sun rising over the snow in the background. The quiet beauty of the sunrise over the orchids in the snow showed me just how beautiful my life had actually become.

I walked outside and saw the angel on the patio outside my studio. This was an angel given to me by a client I had helped in overcoming a nervous breakdown, chronic fatigue, and a major career crisis. The angel had a little basket with a bird in it. The angel seemed to be holding a basket of snow, and she seemed to be reaching out and showing me the snow, as if it were a gift.

I walked the streets around my neighborhood, carefully crunching my way through the snow and ice. Nobody else was up yet. It was just me and the trees and the snow. The pneumonia had come to make me face my grief.

That morning, in the snow, I felt something huge shifting in my life. I did not know what it was yet. It was as if I had suffered through the pneumonia to clear the grief I had not yet even begun to feel.

Perhaps you have had the same experience of an unexpected illness forcing you to examine your own pain and suffering. In the following chapters, I will provide techniques to help you gain greater understanding of pain and suffering, and how we can develop a better relationship with ourselves through the process of healing.

Chapter 71. Pain and Suffering

"The sickness and the pain, or the anger and the attack, whatever it is the person has done, is really a call for help and an expression of that person's identification with his or her ego."

—Kenneth Wapnick

As they say, pain is inevitable, suffering is optional. We all recognize that on some level. Pain is part of life, and we can either accept that nothing is ever going to be always perfect and get on with it, or carry on whining.

Suffering is your mental experience of what is happening. You could be living in a million-dollar mansion and suffering mightily. Trust me on that one. I had a client once who kept telling me he was worth over $15 million. Then one day he came in and said, "The stock market is down. Can you give me a discount?" To someone living in poverty, that may sound ludicrous, but it's true.

One of my friends who lives in London went to visit Africa a few years ago. She came back home and had trouble working. "Catherine," she said, "the people there had so little. Children would follow me down the street begging for the smallest amount of money. I had trouble coming back home and dealing with my clients here in the city. I had trouble wrapping my head around why they were suffering so much when we have so much."

Suffering is a measure of just how much you are resisting what is happening in your life. Once again, if you recognize that it is all God, then it is all good, even if you have not yet figured out the blessing in your challenges.

If I am doing a healing, I will separate the issues of pain and suffering. I will do a healing for pain. And I will do another healing for suffering. They are, in fact, two separate issues. If you look at your patterns of suffering, what you will notice is that there will be a common thread behind it. Listen closely to yourself. There will be a common story.

If you pick up the story and examine it carefully, then you have the opportunity to stop projecting that suffering out into the world. You may notice that your suffering even has a common rhythm to it. For example, you may notice that you start getting upset every Monday night, or Saturday morning, or whatever.

If you have been experiencing a lot of suffering, sit with yourself and listen carefully to the story behind it. It may go something like this:

- "I never get enough."
- "Nobody likes me."
- "Everybody abuses me."
- "Life just sucks."
- "All men/women always do...."

You may never have recognized the story behind the suffering, but it will be there. It may even help you to write it down. You may think that the suffering is caused by something out there—your boss, the economy, your mother/father/childhood, whatever—but, trust me, the answers are all in there, inside of you.

Then notice if there is a rhythm or pattern to your suffering. Your pattern may be bigger than getting set off at a particular day of the week or time of day. Say you always get sick in the winter. Or every Christmas. Or every Easter. See if you can get a calendar out and track it: when it happens, how long it lasts. And notice, if you looked at the recent challenges you have had, if there is a common theme. If it were a piece of music, it would have a certain melody. If it were a lecture, it would have a point to get across. There would be a message.

Chapter 72. The Message of Your Suffering

"Out of suffering have emerged the strongest souls;
the most massive characters are seared with scars."

—Khalil Gibran

If you were going to talk to your suffering, you could start by finding out where you are holding it in your body. You could be holding your suffering anywhere—in an organ, in a bone. It could be in an acupuncture meridian (which would continually keep that meridian firing out of balance), in a chakra, in your breath, or lungs and intercostal muscles (a biggie, as when we go into fight or flight responses, our breathing shuts down and we freeze up in the muscles that help us breathe).

You could well be holding your suffering in your emotional body, which you will probably be experiencing as a constant feeling of pain.

You could be holding that suffering in your mind, such as a belief that the world is a mess, that things are going wrong or that you are actually getting the short end of the stick.

Even your beautiful soul could be suffering. You could be walking around as a wounded spirit, attracting other wounded spirits who serve to confirm for you that your experience of a horrible life must in fact be what is actually happening.

Find out where you are holding your suffering. Ask your angels. Do an intuitive reading. Find out the level where you are holding your suffering and clear it at that level. Then you can truly be done.

Chapter 73. Suffering Meditation

"Oh sad No More! Oh sweet No more!
Oh strange No more!
By a mossed brookbank on a stone
I smelt a wildweed-flower alone;
There was a ringing in my ears,
And both my eyes gushed out with tears."

—Alfred Lord Tennyson

Lie down in a comfortable location. Get as totally relaxed as possible. Clear your energy.

Call in your angels and spiritual guides to help you. Say a prayer and ask to be shown where you are holding your suffering. Here is a prayer you can start with:

Mother/Father/God/Universal Source,
  Thank you so much for my life.
  Thank you for all you have been giving me.
  Thank you for all the love and support I am currently experiencing.
  For some reason, I have been suffering.

*Please show me where I am holding my suffering
so that I may experience healing now.
Thank you. Amen.*

With your eyes shut, look, listen, and feel. You may think you know where you are suffering. You may think you are suffering in an obvious place that has been hurting, but your answer could possibly surprise you.

When you find your suffering, notice it. Get curious about it. Does it have a weight? Does it have a color? Does it have a feeling behind it? Go as deeply into the feeling as you can.

And here is a hint: the deeper you go into the feeling, the more you actually heal it. Breathe into it. Look at it. Allow yourself to get curious. Ironically, be almost objective, but at the same time get as close as you can go into what it actually feels like.

Years ago, I went to the dentist for a routine checkup. While I was there, he told me I needed caps on two of my lower teeth. When I went to pay for my appointment, the receptionist told me that if I came back the next day to get my teeth capped, that they would give me a discount.

I realized I needed to face the music (as one of my clients once said, "But is it country music?"), so I signed up to come back the next day. The dentist drilled away on my teeth. Somehow in doing so he damaged the nerves in my teeth, jaw, and face.

Next came three of the most painful months in my life. I suffered so much, I could hardly believe myself. I went to the health food store to find a homeopathic to help me. I stood in front of the row of remedies and muscle tested myself. I picked up the one I needed and read the information about it. "For when your teeth feel so bad, you feel like screaming," it said. That would be the one!

Meanwhile, I had signed up for two seminars in New York City that I had already paid for. I had my hotel room booked. I really wanted to learn the information, and I wanted my brain to work properly, so I didn't take any pain reliever stronger than an aspirin so I could think straight and remember clearly. Being in a state of pain and suffering is definitely an energy-consuming experience.

I don't remember all that much about those two seminars, other than the fact that I was trying really hard. I showed up at every class exactly on time. On my way home from the second class, I called the dentist's office. I ended up having to have two emergency root canals. My brother, a doctor, was the one who diagnosed the problem.

I had trigeminal neuralgia, which is the most painful affliction described in the medical literature. During this time, I used the technique of breathing into my suffering and feeling my feelings. I would go as deeply as I could into the experience.

I also asked a fellow healer for insight. "You are dropping all your genetic programming on all the levels all at one time," she told me.

"Oh!" I said. "No wonder that is so painful!"

"Now you will be in choice," she said to me. "You get to decide for yourself how to move forward."

Sometimes when we are in pain, we are releasing at very deep levels.

Chapter 74. Genomes, Genetics, and Family History

"I refuse to join any club that would have me as a member."

—Groucho Marx

It turned out that both my father and paternal grandmother had also suffered from trigeminal neuralgia. Even though I did not know beforehand that this had been the case, I found myself living out a very painful family pattern and it had come down to me to clear it. Many of the things that we go through as human beings come through our biological lineage—even issues that don't seem like they would be genetic.

One client came to me for female problems. It turned out that all the women in her family had hysterectomies around their mid-thirties.

This is where genomes come in. A *genome* is a

thought pattern you inherited either consciously or unconsciously from your ancestors, beginning with either your mother or father, grandmothers or grandfathers. It could be as simple as, "In your thirties, you are going to get _____ (fill in the blank—a hysterectomy, cancer, a heart attack, what have you) because that is what everybody in the family gets." You may or may not be consciously aware of genomes or of just how much these genetic thought patterns are affecting you.

A genome could be manifesting in your physical health, but it could also be affecting literally any other aspect of your life. Another example of a genome is, "All the women in the family are successful, but the men, not so much." Or, "Nobody in our family has ever amounted to anything." Or, "You are probably going to end up looking like your Aunt Sally because all the women in the family end up with big hips." One of my personal favorites is, "Everybody in the family is crazy!"

One way to identify whether genomes are holding you back is by recalling the stories that you heard while growing up.

Take out a sheet of paper and write down every negative message you can ever remember being given about health, happiness, or personal success. This may take a while!

If possible, see if you can remember who told you each story, as the genome could have originated with your mother, your father, or both, or your grandmother or grandfather and the stories they told you could possibly carry back many generations.

If I am doing a healing to clear a genome for a client, I identify the thought pattern and then use kinesiology to trace the lineage back through multiple generations until I find the ancestor with whom that thought had originated.

If you were given repeated messages that people in your family have particular difficulties being healthy, happy, or successful, then you will want to do a healing to clear those genetic thought patterns so that you can clear them all the way through your cellular level.

You could also be participating in a *miasm*, which is more of a global or cultural thought pattern. A good example of a miasm is, "You have to go on a diet in order to lose weight." Another miasm is, "We are experiencing a global recession."

You can participate in a negative thought pattern or not, but the first step is to recognize that you are actually acting out stories that did not orginate with you.

You may be consciously aware of genetics, your DNA. You could have a family history of heart disease, for example. I know of one woman who worked very hard to avoid her family history of heart disease. She exercised daily, kept her weight under control, took a ton of nutritional supplements, worked with her doctor to perform heart stress tests regularly to monitor her situation and still ended up with heart disease. Although she had followed sound advice about her physical health, she had not cleared the core issues. Many of the issues we carry forward are not really our fault, per se; they are just a consequence of being born a human.

Many of my more aware clients have done the inner work of thinking and feeling their way through their issues and taking the actions necessary to live healthy, happy, and successful lifes but still not come to any resolution. This can be a great source of frustration if you have been trying very hard but don't seem to be getting anywhere. And that may be because your issues didn't actually start with you. If this is the case with you, then you may want to clear at a deeper level.

One of my favorite ways to clear genomes and genetic issues is to do what is called a seven-generation healing. You begin with yourself and ask for a healing on all levels. Then you ask for guidance about whether to ask for assistance from your maternal line or your paternal line. Then, stepping back to either your father or mother, you ask for guidance and assistance.

These people may be alive or dead; it really doesn't matter. You are having a soul-to-soul communication. On that level, everyone is everywhere always present.

You step back from one generation to the next, continuing to ask for healing.

One of my clients was a university professor. A very dignified gentleman, he had to walk with a cane due to unrelenting gout. Although he learned a lot from me about his nutrition, the thing that actually healed him completely was walking back through his ancestry and asking his previous seven generations for divine assistance.

At the time we did the healing, this very learned

gentleman wept. He was surprised to learn he was actually able to hear each ancestor speaking to him. The experience was totally outside his realm of previous experience. He had thought his ancestors were all long gone and that he was now on his own. He was wrong.

Another way to clear genomes and miasms that did not originate with us is by doing a karmic clearing. Karma can be thought of as results, good or bad, that you are carrying forward.

I use kinesiology to determine the pattern to be cleared and then muscle test to make sure you are ready, willing, and able to clear that pattern now. You could be holding a pattern on a mental level. That would be showing up in repeated thoughts either conscious or subconscious. You could be holding your pattern in your DNA, which means you are carrying forward through your genetic heritage.

Or you could also have a karmic contract with another person. Your soul may have agreed to help another soul, or vice versa. Karmic contracts can either be one way or mutual. Either way, you can do a healing and be complete with the pain and suffering.

Time and again, I have seen a person who a client thought was their worst enemy in this lifetime was, in fact, on the soul level their very best friend. This could be the person forcing you to grow, allowing you to face your greatest fears and to find the strength inside yourself that you did not know was there all along.

And finally, you could be carrying this karma through the core of your soul, which means you have been suffering with this pattern for a very long time, so that you are carrying the energy of this negativity not just in your physical body but all the way through to your soul level. Needless to say, this is the most painful way to carry karma and one of the most powerful places from which to heal.

Chapter 75. There Is No Time, There Is No Space; It's All One Energy

"It is only when we have the courage to face things exactly as they are, without any self-deception or illusion, that a light will develop out of events, by which the path to success may be recognized."

—I Ching

Sometimes my clients ask me how I know what I know. I have had clients in Australia, and I am telling them deep insights all about themselves, and then I am sharing about their mother, who I have also never seen, laid my hands on, or ever communicated with in any physical way. How could it be that a person in another continent can know all about you, be actually accurate, and be able to help you? It sounds fantastic and ridiculous.

As you practice opening your psychic gifts and talking to your angels, you will be connecting to universal energy. One of the first things to understand is that there is no such thing as time or space. It's all just one energy. And, as I have been saying, it's all God, and therefore it's all good.

Time and space are really only conveniences of awareness. They help us to keep things in some semblance of order. It's like your spice cabinet. Where is the salt? Where is the pepper? Whatever happened to the rosemary; surely there is some in there somewhere?

What an effort it is to keep even your sock drawer in some semblance of order, where you can separate the black ones from the brown ones!

For example, you could take a car trip through Arizona. As you are driving along, it could seem like you are going from one place to another and, as you are driving along, you are having different experiences. But it's all just Arizona.

Change your understanding about what reality is, and then you will be able to know a lot more. And it's fun.

CHAPTER 76. THERE ARE ONLY FOUR PROBLEMS, EVER

"If you can't explain it simply, you don't understand it well enough."

—ALBERT EINSTEIN

I am a simple person and I like to keep things simple. I work out of my home. I like to work with Belle—or should I say she has decided already that she is working with me. I like not to work too hard. I only keep as many orchids in my studio as I can actually take care of easily.

I just recently put down drought-resistant perennials in my front yard because it seemed too complicated and expensive to have to reseed my grass every year, and to constantly pour on chemicals and water. Being a simple-minded person, I like to keep my work simple.

Even though I have studied all this information

about intuition and about every aspect of healing work that I could put my hands on, when it comes to working with what I call actual humans, the simpler the better, I feel.

So, the way I see it, there are only four problems, ever. These four problems are:

- **Blocks:** Impediments to change. A block can be physical, energetic, emotional, mental, or spiritual.
- **Congestion:** An accumulation, clogging, or overcrowding of energy preventing change. Congestion may be either physical, energetic, emotional, mental, or spiritual.
- **Resistance:** Lack of willingness. Your ego is opposing the process of change. This is primarily emotional or mental.
- **Interference:** A force outside yourself is preventing change. This is actually the least likely problem, as we are always in charge of our own lives, whether or not we choose to accept responsibility for our own power.

So, if you are experiencing literally any challenge in any aspect of your life, you can ask your guidance if you have a block, congestion, resistance, interference, or some combination of the above. Sometimes in life, our issues can appear completely overwhelming. It may take you hours just to tell your story, to explain all the gnarly details, and in the process you may become very emotionally overwhelmed and unable to think clearly enough to see your way out of your challenges.

You can use the power of your intuition to

understand the root issues of what is going on, and that can go a long way to helping you know what you can actually do to get better. Blocks, congestion, resistance, and interference all feel and look very different when perceived through the power of your intuition.

Each of the four problems will require a different solution. If you ask guidance to simplify any issue for you, the solutions will become self-evident.

Chapter 77. Blocks

"Frisbeetarianism is the belief that when you die, your soul goes up on the roof and gets stuck."

—George Carlin

A block happened one time when a hurricane hit my yard. A tree that had been happily living just outside my studio—one so big you couldn't put your arms all the way around it—fell down across the side street beside my house. I was upstairs when it happened. It took just a few seconds for this humongous tree to come crashing down. Fortunately, no one was driving on the side street. And, thankfully, the tree did not fall on my house. It fell away from my house. The tree blocked the side street. No cars could get by. That is a good example of a block.

Energetically speaking, a block is something that is stuck and not moving. A block could also be something that you are not able to see. In kinesiology, we talk about what is called the Johari window. There are things you know about that other people also know. This is also called your arena.

Let's say that you know your name is Joe. Other people would probably know that also. That falls into the category of what you know about you that other people know also.

Then there are things that you know that other people don't know about you. You know what happened when you were four years old. Other people weren't there, so they don't know what happened to you when you were four.

This is precisely why when other people look at you and try to figure out why you do what you do they usually really have no idea.

For example, one of the most profound healings I ever experienced was about sitting in a chair. I was studying healing with Sue Maes, an extraordinary kinesiologist and medical intuitive. Sue asked for a volunteer; she wanted to teach what we all thought was a relatively simple technique, a postural stress release, which is a technique to release stress held in the body around simple, everyday activities, such as sitting in a chair or driving a car.

Like many people, I don't like sitting for long periods of time, so I volunteered to be the demo model. Even though I have always been an avid learner, if I went to a class, I would rather be sitting on the floor, pacing the room, or lying with my legs against the wall rather than sitting in a chair. No doubt this was distracting and uncomfortable for everyone else, teacher and other students alike, but up until that point, I just couldn't keep still sitting in a chair.

As soon as Sue began the postural stress release, I remembered being a teenage girl in a special program for exceptional high school science students of Savannah, Georgia, where I grew up. I was one of only two girls sitting in a room full of boys when I realized that my period had started. I was sitting in the front row and was afraid to stand up. When I stood up, I was mortified to see blood all over the seat of the chair. When I went home, I announced to my parents I was so embarrassed that I never wanted to return to the science program. My father responded by beating me. I went back to the science program every week that followed, even though I remained deeply humiliated. During the healing that Sue guided me through, I cried, wept, and trembled; it was finally safe for my body to release the trauma I had experienced sitting in that chair and all that followed as a result.

Your history is like your file cabinet. You yourself may not even consciously recall everything that has happened to you, but every cell in your body actually does.

Other people have a totally different history and, therefore, a totally different file cabinet.

When you do something, other people may go into their own history, their own file cabinet, and say to themselves, "I would never do that," or, "I would not have done it that way." This is a major cause of misunderstandings between people; they go into their own filing cabinets to try to understand, and then project their own history and experience onto others. But they don't know your history, they don't have your filing cabinet, and they really have no clue.

This is why it is always a big mistake to judge other people. Even if we think we know, we really actually do not have 100 percent of all the information about why other people make the choices that they make. It's their journey.

Then there are things that other people know about you that you don't know. Let's say you went to the bathroom and have toilet paper accidentally tacked to your shoe. A kind soul could point that out before you had the opportunity to make more of a fool out of yourself. This is your blind spot.

Then there is a last, really juicy window. It's the window that you don't know about yourself that other people don't know about you. This is the really juicy window because it probably holds the issues that you have not been able to see in yourself and, therefore, what you haven't been able to deal with. You didn't see it, you didn't know it and, therefore, nothing was done about it.

I say this is the juicy window because this is the place where you can potentially make the greatest shift in your personal healing. It's the unknown. When you bring the light of awareness to these unknown places in yourself, your life, you have the opportunity to make big changes. Even intuitive people have these hidden places. It's not the same as your shadow self; it's literally the places where you just haven't looked, where you have no idea.

One time I realized I had actually fallen in love

with another person. When I realized it, I felt like an idiot. How could I have not have seen that? It's because everybody has an unknown window. And that is where we are blocked.

Working with a kinesiologist, medical intuitive, therapist, or other objective, outside party can be very helpful here as you can locate parts of yourself and do something about them. That would be like a runner suddenly discovering the resources to shave another several seconds off his or her sprint.

If you look at awareness objectively, you can only see so much at a certain time because you are only seeing reality from your current viewpoint. When you can see a bigger picture, you can see your blocks, and you can do something about them.

CHAPTER 78. CONGESTION

"If they'd lower the taxes and get rid of the smog and clean up the traffic mess, I really believe I'd settle here until the next earthquake."

—GROUCHO MARX

When you use the power of your intuition, you will find that energetically, congestion feels overfilled or crowded with excessive accumulation. You can have congestion in your home. You can have congestion in your body. You can really have congestion everywhere. It is not uncommon for me to tell a new client, "Go home and clean up even just one room in your house."

If you are congested in your large intestine acupuncture meridian, you will have trouble letting go. If you have trouble letting go in one place, you will have trouble letting go everywhere. As above, so below.

One of the major aspects of feng shui (see chapter

forty-four) is about removing congested energy. When the energy in your home or office space is flowing freely, you can be physically healthy, mentally calm, peaceful, and more productive.

Understanding more about feng shui has made me more attentive to the simple practice of cleaning up. Vacuuming. Dusting. Throwing things away. Giving old, unused items to Goodwill.

In the body, congestion comes in the form of clogged arteries, plaque in the brain, a liver that doesn't work right, a digestive system that is sluggish, a lymph system that doesn't move, a circulatory system that is running slowly. All this adds up to fatigue and feeling yucky (that's a scientific term, by the way).

You can clear congestion in the body by eating very clean foods, like lots of fruits and vegetables, and moving your energy through healthy exercise.

Mentally, congestion may show up as confusion. We ask twenty different people for their opinions, rather than simply asking for guidance about which step will lead to our highest good.

One time I went to the paint store and spent a week trying to determine which shade of grey to paint my office. I put an app on my iPhone and would drive myself nuts; I spent hours comparing the different hues and holding them up to the wall at different times of the day to see how the color reflected in various lights. We may read five different news sources online, cluttering our heads with the facts and figures about what is supposedly going on in the news, rather than just feeling the energy of the day and following the course of least resistance. It is very easy to get swept up in the drama of other people's opinions and the turmoil of our own reactions.

You can clear the congestion mentally simply by taking time throughout the day to get quiet. Go for a walk in nature, stop talking, cease the ingestion of useless but seemingly important information. Stop allowing yourself to be programmed outside yourself and be your own channel.

CHAPTER 79. RESISTANCE

"I was not naturally talented. I didn't sing, dance or act, though working around that minor detail made me inventive."

—STEVE MARTIN

This one is a biggie. Earlier in this book, I talked about the importance of willingness. You can resist anything—even good ideas, or things that you know would be helpful for you, make you more money, or make you happier and healthier. Resistance is all about keeping things the same in a vain effort to try to feel safer. The trouble is, one of the few things that you can actually bet your money on is change. Life begins at the end of your comfort zone.

The entire vibration of the planet is speeding up. So when we go into resistance, we are putting up a futile attempt to maintain our small existence. Even if you are completely uncomfortable with your status quo, it's what you have grown accustomed to.

Being human, I understand all about resistance. I can look outside the window of my studio at practically any season. In the autumn, when the leaves turn and start to fall when the wind breaks, I see the shiny yellow and gold patterns glittering through the sky. *This the most beautiful time of year,* I think. In my mind, I want to hold onto it. I want the view always to look the same.

Then the winter comes. Suddenly, I can see deep into the trees across the street. The sunlight comes through in a different way. Everything feels quiet. *I love this the best,* I think. And then we have one or two snowstorms every year, like frosting on the cake and, wow, it all seems totally magical.

I am still hanging onto my view of this beauty and then, all of a sudden, spring breaks, the azaleas bloom all at once, there is a riot of light pink and hot pink, and the blooms of the azaleas surround the angel outside my studio like a halo of appreciation.

Oh my gosh, I think, *I wish the azaleas would bloom like this all year.*

Then the rain comes, dashes the blossoms to the ground, the flowers go away, and the summer begins. The euphorbia and double begonias around my blue jar fountain spill over the flowerbed. The purple jade flowers and petunias trail over the wall to my studio like a welcome banner to all who come to see me.

My gardener, Gabe, and I are amazed at how this one flowerbed goes bonkers. We don't even fertilize the flowers there; they just are so happy and grow all over each other like a prize-winning garden you might see in a botanical garden someplace.

Every season seems more beautiful than the next. When I try to resist the advent of a new season, I remind myself about resistance. I remind myself that I am safe through all the changes.

You can resist even beauty in your life. But it's all God, so it's all good.

Chapter 80. Interference

"You don't drown by falling in the water; you drown by staying there."

—Edwin Louis Cole

People usually put a lot of weight into interference, as though what is wrong with us must be the fault of other people or outside forces. This is true sometimes, but it is not usually the case.

I had a mother-in-law who visited me once. She told me she had a great idea about how to rearrange my living room. She moved all the furniture to exactly how she liked it. I allowed her to have her interference. Then, once she was gone, I moved everything back to where I liked it.

Interference, when it really is a problem, is usually with things that you have no conscious awareness of, such as with sensitivity to electromagnetic radiation.

On the Isle of Gigha in Scotland, I visited my friend Don Dennis, who raises orchids and develops flower essences from them. Because Don knew that I was a medical intuitive and, therefore, highly sensitive to energies, he put me in the room that was the most sheltered from the high-frequency cell towers that the government of the United Kingdom had erected. He said that many of the cell towers were affecting peoples' ability to sleep well.

Even though I was exhausted from my trip, and even though I took steps to protect myself from EMFs, I still had trouble sleeping and felt sleep deprived most of the trip. Geopathic stress is a good example of interference.

Many people are not aware of how much their health and energy levels are affected by factors in their environment that go way beyond the parameters of feng shui. War, for example, or the nuclear meltdown at Chernobyl, can also be contributing environmental factors.

I clear geopathic stress in my healing work. You would be surprised how so many factors in our everyday, modern existence—TV, radio waves, cellphone towers, waste treatment plants, radiation, airplane noises—are affecting you at the cellular levels. You would be even more surprised at others, such as the shapes of buildings, for example, or underground streams.

I once worked with a young woman who was an orphan adopted from Romania. Literally every time I worked with her, her system showed she was reacting to geopathic stress. And when I checked to see what that geopathic stress was, the answer was "atomic bomb." Even though my client was a very young child at the time of the meltdown at Chernobyl, her mind/body/soul had interpreted the accident as if an atomic bomb had gone off nearby.

It took us a while to get her system out of chronic stress; she had been in survival mode her for most of her life, even though she had been adopted into a very loving family.

The combined total of geopathic stress in urban areas like New York City is quite extreme, but you could still be experiencing geopathic stress on a quiet mountaintop. You could still be reacting to wind or thunder or major earth changes.

CHAPTER 81. BE STRONG ENOUGH TO HANDLE YOUR SENSITIVITY

> "Intuition is the supra-logic that cuts out all the routine processes of thought and leaps straight from the problem to the answer."
>
> —ROBERT GRAVES

If you are reading this book, you may realize you have a sensitive nature wrapped around your psychic gifts. If you do, then I strongly encourage you to become strong enough to handle your sensitivity.

Many highly sensitive people have trouble functioning in everyday life. They may even wear their sensitivity as a badge of honor. I once attended a lecture of a well-known medical intuitive. She proudly stated that she was writing another book and was so ungrounded that she was not sure she could speak in front of an audience. She talked about walking into the wrong hotel room and being rude to the people who were occupying the room, and getting lost in her neighborhood grocery store. Being so sensitive that you can't function in the world is not a good thing. Once again, heal thyself first. Learn to ground yourself.

Grounding is incredibly important because it keeps you real, it keeps you in the here and now, and it helps you to relate to ordinary people.

I clean my own house. I exercise regularly. I knew a long time ago that, because of my abilities, I had to make a major effort to connect to my physical body. It was a lot easier for me to disconnect and be someplace else. In fact, I don't even have to shut my eyes for my mind or soul to go someplace else. It's just part of the gift.

I regularly visit another healer who does hands-on healing with me. She tells me that when she first started working with me years ago, she could not find me.

I love to garden because it helps me connect to the earth. I play with my dog and visit with my friends. Knitting and beading help me stay in the here and now in a very pleasant way.

Signs that you are way too sensitive include not being able to handle public transportation or riding in a car. I had trouble riding in cars for years. I have done so many healings on that issue, I can't even count them all. The root of it was that I could literally feel the energies of all the other cars, all the people in them, what they were thinking and not thinking, what they were aware of and not aware of. And, yet, I live in Atlanta, a city of many interstates. I have to be able to get across town without losing my mind.

Grounding will make your life easier and also make it easier for other people to be around you. Activities that ground you are practical, everyday tasks that slow you down to the earth vibration, like walking barefoot, cleaning, cooking, gardening, and exercising your physical body.

Also, if you have many environmental or food sensitivities, your entire nervous system is too sensitive. I recommend working through all that before taking on the energies of working with clients yourself.

You can do a gut-healing program to strengthen the immune system in your gastrointestinal tract, and use kinesiology to clear your sensitivities so that you can eat and live with other people.

If you are not able to handle the energy in your own life very well, you won't be able to handle the energies you pick up from other people.

At one point, I was sensitive or allergic to every food tested except Brazil nuts and lentils. Try eating that for a diet! I healed my digestive system and brought my level of sensitivity down.

One thing that helps you to handle your sensitivity is to learn what you personally need to do to keep your energy protected. There are many different techniques. Some of the simplest include wearing purple bracelets on your wrists when you do any kind of hands-on healing, which prevents you from taking on the energies of other people.

We had a drought one summer in Atlanta, and I could literally feel all the trees and shrubs dying. I couldn't do anything about it; it was not like I could go around watering all the trees and shrubs in my neighborhood!

It is helpful to remember that all living beings have free will, even trees and shrubs. Each of us has a choice about what we choose to experience. Choose to be in your body, healthy and happy, and you will go a long way toward radiating that peace and joy to others.

Chapter 82. Why Using Your Intuition For Health Is Important Now

"It is through science that we prove, but through intuition that we discover."

—Henri Poincare

We live in a time of scarce medical resources. Getting sick is very expensive. According to the *American Journal of Medicine*, 60 percent of bankruptcies are now driven by health care costs.

One of my long-term clients, a bankruptcy attorney, told me of the pain she experiences watching average, middle-class people filing bankruptcy after experiencing a major illness.

My father and brother are both medical doctors. I honor their profession. I also listen to their experiences, including how challenging it is now to run a medical practice.

My brother is an ophthalmologist. Most of his

clients are cataract patients, and are on Medicare. He says that makes him a de facto government employee, even though he runs his own surgery center.

You can be super astute and a great doctor, run your own business and, still, bureaucrats, who do not necessarily have the best interests of you or your patients in mind, boss you around. The government is constantly driving him crazy with all the changes of rules and regulations.

With the cost of health care going up, people are looking for quick, easy, and cost-effective solutions. They want to know what will work. This is where medical intuitive work comes in.

The average interaction between a patient and a general physician lasts an average of 18.7 minutes, according to the *Annals of Family Medicine*. Research shows that shorter visits result in lower patient satisfaction and possibly poorer quality of care.

I always joke that it doesn't take that long to figure out what is wrong with someone. What takes time is the process of awakening—helping you to see the many ways you can make yourself better, even to realize that it is possible to get better, as so many people who come to me have lost hope.

The average length of one of my sessions is ninety minutes. I take the time to listen and to explain. One of my gifts is being able to empower you to find not only the deeper meaning behind your illness, but also what will actually work to make you better.

Using your intuitive gifts to tune into your own health and the health of other people may speed up, simplify, and lower the cost of the entire process.

CHAPTER 83: LETTING GO

"People travel to wonder at the height of the mountains, at the huge waves of the seas, at the long course of the rivers, at the vast compass of the ocean, at the circular motion of the stars, and yet they pass by themselves without wondering."

—St. Augustine

Angels speak to us in many funny ways. They speak directly to us. They light our paths at dawn. They show us images in our mind's eye of the route that would be better to take. They help us to stop what we are doing and pay attention. Often the angels in our lives are real people. Or they can even be our pets. If we stop and pay attention, the angels may even be birds we can't exactly see singing to us from a faraway bush.

Everywhere, in all creation, we are lifted up, loved, and supported. If I am doing a medical intuitive reading, even if you are asking me about your physical body, I am communicating with you soul to soul. This is sacred communication—nothing to be afraid of.

Spirit only gives you what you need to know right now. Spirit only gives you what you need in this moment, what you can handle, and what your angels know you can handle. Some of the messages your angels and soul will give me are quite simple:

"Learn to love yourself," "Be happy," or "All is well."

Once, a good friend came to me with a pain in her right side. I told her it was her liver. "Detox immediately," I advised her, checking with her body for the precise steps she needed. About six weeks later, she came back. The same pain was on her right side. "You're detoxing?" I asked her.

"I ran out," she replied.

I asked Spirit what needed to be done. It was a Friday afternoon: the end of the day at end of the week. "Go to the doctor first thing Monday morning," I recommended. "There is nothing else any alternative practitioner can do for you."

She protested. The test was going to be very expensive, about $1,500. I shrugged my shoulders. I got my friend to get her doctor on the phone while she was in my office. I made sure she had made the appointment. She went to the doctor on Monday and did the test. It was liver cancer. About the time I had told her about her liver, a medical practitioner had run a lab test that yielded the same result. However, my friend did not get the information for some reason. I had told her, but she didn't get the information from the doctor. It was as if her own soul didn't want to get the message from anybody.

When she finally got the diagnosis of liver cancer, I felt crushed. I love my friend. I love all my clients. The thought that I might lose her—that we all might lose her—pained me greatly. I went into soul searching and turned to a friend who is a long-time healer and mentor.

"Spirit only tells you what you are supposed to hear. If you had gotten the diagnosis of cancer, you would have healed her, and that is not her path," she said.

In cancer, the energy in the body is pulled up. There could even be holes. I had gotten my friend to go immediately to the doctor. I had gotten that right.

A few weeks later, I spoke to my friend for about an hour. She was angry. She was also ambivalent. She told me the doctors said that if she didn't do anything, she would have about sixty to ninety days left.

I remembered what my friend the healer said to me: if I had gotten the message about the cancer that I would have healed her, and that was not her path. I had put a tremendous amount of energy into my friend. I had organized a prayer circle for her the year before. I had made jewelry and blessed it with Reiki. And, most of all, I wanted to see her feeling well and being happy. But that was not her path. We have to honor the path of each individual and realize that death itself is only a transition.

My friend appeared to others to be putting up a good fight. Several weeks after our last phone conversation, her spirit came to me and said goodbye.

I understood completely. It was another six weeks or so before she made her actual transition.

The form in which you choose to make your passing may give the opportunity to say goodbye. I think my friend needed to take her time to say goodbye, even though she had been ready for some time.

CHAPTER 84. THE PRIVILEGE TO BE TOGETHER IN THIS TIME AND SPACE

"When the doors of perception are cleansed man will see things as they truly are, infinite."

—WILLIAM BLAKE

The week my grandfather died, I was determined for him not to die alone. At that point, he was bedridden in a nursing home. My grandmother had passed earlier. He lay in bed, barely breathing, his dear, sweet face covered in sweat. I sat beside him and read the Bible aloud. I took the week off to be with him every second that I could. I held his hand. He had been one of the true loves of my life and had always been kind to me.

I read aloud and also silently, but still nothing happened. He lay in bed with no change. Finally, one morning, he seemed to awake. He said, "I went through the doorway." But that was it. I never heard him speak ever again. I continued to read the Bible to him.

Although my grandfather, a chemist and inventor, was as a good a soul as you will ever meet, it came to my attention in later years that he was not a believer. He told me at the time that he had grown up in a German immigrant community down in Texas. He was trained as a scientist. He revered the scientific method. To him, the Bible was "just a bunch of fairy tales," he told me.

When I heard that my grandfather was an agnostic, I was perplexed about what to do. I remembered that for about sixty years my grandmother had gone to church, but she had always gone alone.

A friend put things into some perspective. "Don't shake the rock that is his firm foundation now." But, at his end, in my time of turmoil, I turned to my own foundation. As I sat there reading to him, day after day, it occurred to me that as much as I did not want my grandfather to die alone, his soul wanted to spare me his transition. I realized that it was his time to go, and as long as I was there, that he wasn't going anywhere. So I left.

Within two days, he passed away. At the end, his epitaph reassured me. He had written something very short, being a man of few words. He let it be known that in the expanse of the universe, in all of time and space, he felt blessed to have been with my grandmother. And that was all.

As much as we all want to be healthy and happy, and as much as we want that state for our friends and loved ones, we have to learn to let them go.

I let my friend go. I let my grandfather go. And their passings informed me and my work that this world is a glorious place, and that we are all privileged to share this joyous experience.

I bless all those who choose to be healthier and happier. I also allow each soul to make his or her own choice and to leave when it is the time to do so. As we mark the passing of our loved ones, let us all remember how precious it is to have been born a human in this time and in this space.

APPENDIX:

THE CHAKRAS
AND THEIR ASSOCIATIONS

The Chakras and Their Associations

Although much has been written about the chakras by many other authors, I would like to provide my perspective from teaching about these energy centers and also healing them for many years.

First, it is very helpful to understand the way that energy flows through your body. Energy enters your body through the crown of your head. There is a vertical electrical current, your hara line, that runs from above the crown of your head through your physical body down into the center of the Earth.

Your hara line feeds energy into vortexes of energy called chakras. There are seven major chakras, and depending on who you listen to, countless others. I have studied with other healers who believe you have as many as twenty-seven chakras extending well above your head, connecting you into the cosmos.

The chakras feed energy into your acupuncture meridians. Your acupuncture meridians feed energy into your organs. And, finally, your organs feed energy into your muscles.

So, if you have a health problem or you are not feeling as happy as you could be, the question becomes where along this complex system your energy may not be flowing as efficiently as it could. Physical illness may shut down your chakras, but so may any emotional, mental, or spiritual issue. If your chakras are not functioning properly, they may literally be clogged with old energy and information that you have subconsciously held on to.

As an energy healer, I am able to clean out this old energy and rebuild your chakra. These energy centers may be spinning backward, as opposed to spinning clockwise, which is what happens when we are mentally, emotionally, and physically healthy.

On the other hand, when your hara line is open, you are connected to the Earth and to the divine at the same time, your chakras are all open and balanced, you will feel both grounded and divinely guided, healthy and happy, all in an effortless way.

I believe that keeping your energy system open and healthy is essential for receiving intuitive information, because each chakra allows us to process energy and information of high value.

The following information comes from a class I have taught for many years about how to heal your chakras.

1st Chakra, Muladhara, Root Chakra

Purpose: our foundation

- Issues associated with 1st chakra:
- Roots
- Grounding
- Trust
- Health
- Home
- Family
- Appropriate boundaries
- Prosperity
- Courage
- Vitality
- Self-confidence
- Survival
- Money
- Seat of kundalini

If your 1st chakra is deficient, you may experience:
- Major illness or injury
- Disconnection from the body
- Fretful, anxious, can't settle down
- Poor focus, poor discipline
- Financial problems
- Poor boundaries
- Chronic disorganization

If your 1st chakra is excessive, you may experience:
- Hoarding
- Overeating
- Greed
- Fear of change, addiction to security
- Rigid boundaries

Color: Red

Glands: Adrenals

Developmental age:
2nd trimester in the womb to 12 months

Balanced characteristics:
- Good health
- Vitality
- Well grounded
- Comfortable in your body
- Sense of trust in the world
- Feeling safe and secure
- Able to relax and be still
- Stable
- Prosperous
- Right livelihood

Physical malfunctions:
- Disorders of the bowel, anus, digestive system
- Adrenal burnout
- Disorders of the solid parts of the body: bones, teeth
- Issues with feet, legs, knees, base of spine,

buttocks, hips
- Eating disorders
- Frequent illness
- Obesity

Affirmations that support your 1st chakra:
- I have a right to be here
- I am safe
- I love my body and trust its wisdom
- I live a life of abundance
- I choose to be here in this body in this lifetime
- I love my life
- I am meaningfully connected to my family
- I draw on my family for love and support
- I honor my connections to my tribe and transcend them
- I have plenty of money now
- I nurture my connection with nature

To heal wounds of your 1st chakra:
- Get hugged or held
- Create good bedding to you feel safe and comfortable as you sleep
- Garden
- Cook
- Take a walk
- Go barefoot
- Have a picnic
- Physical exercise
- Lots of touch, massage
- Reconnect with your body
- Look at your earliest childhood relationship to

your mother
- Eat meat, proteins, red fruits and red vegetables
- Resolve old family conflicts
- Get out of survival mode and feel prosperous

Sound: Lam, C note

Yoga postures that benefit your 1st chakra:
- Standing poses, especially warrior poses, frog, butterfly, pelvic lifts, bridge, knee to chest, head to knee, seated boat, tortoise, eagle, lotus

2nd Chakra, Svadisthana, Navel Chakra

Purpose: Balanced Power and Sexuality

Issues associated with 2nd chakra:
- Sexuality
- Ability to experience pleasure
- Power
- Creativity
- Intimate relationships
- Desire
- Sexual identity

If the 2nd chakra is deficient:
Rigid physical body and attitudes
- Fear of sex
- Poor social skills
- Denial of pleasure
- Excessive boundaries
- Lack of desire, passion or excitement

- Powerless

If the 2nd chakra is excessive:
- Addiction to sex, drugs or alcohol
- Mood swings
- Excessive sensitivity
- Overpowering, invasion of others
- Emotional codependency
- Obsessive attachments

Color: Orange

Glands: Ovaries, testes

Developmental age: 6 to 24 months

Balanced characteristics:
Graceful movement
- Emotional intelligence
- In your own power
- Comfortable with your own sexuality
- Able to change
- Healthy boundaries
- Emotionally balanced
- Ability to nurture self and others
- Ability to experience pleasure in healthy ways

Physical malfunctions:
- Disorders of the reproductive system
- Menstrual problems
- Sexual dysfunction
- Low back pain, knee trouble

- Lack of flexibility, either physically or emotionally
- Inappropriate appetite (either too much or not enough)

Affirmations
- I have a right to enjoy pleasure
- I accept and celebrate my sexuality
- I deserve to have fun
- I feel comfortable as a man/woman
- My sexuality is sacred
- My life is pleasurable
- I am flexible and go with the flow in life
- I nurture and support all my relationships
- I let go of all past emotional traumas
- I am creative

To heal wounds of your 2nd chakra:
- Give or receive massage
- Take a bath
- Work with your hands
- Swim
- Sit in a rocking chair
- Clean your house
- Feel music
- Inner child work
- Allow your hips to sway when walking
- 12-step programs for addictions
- Develop a healthy hobby just for fun
- Develop healthy boundaries
- Learn how to have healthy intimate relationships

- Honor your femininity/masculinity
- Eat orange fruits and vegetables

Sound: Vam, D note

Yoga postures that benefit your 2nd chakra:
- Forward bends, cobra, sphinx, boat, locust, bow, butterfly, child with knees apart, hip circles, pelvic lifts, hero, spinal twist

3rd Chakra, Manipura, Solar Plexus Chakra

Purpose: Center of psychic feelings

Issues associated with your 3rd chakra:
- Personal identity
- Well balanced energy
- Will power
- Self esteem
- Personal achievement
- Balanced ego

If your 3rd chakra is deficient:
- Low energy
- Weak willed, easily manipulated
- Low self esteem
- Poor digestion
- Victim mentality
- Poor me
- Passive
- Unreliable
- Easily overwhelmed by the thoughts and

feelings of others

If your 3rd chakra is excessive:
- Dominating, controlling, overly aggressive
- Need to be right
- Temper tantrums
- Stubborn
- Type A personality
- Arrogant
- Hyperactive

Color: Yellow

Gland: Pancreas

Development age: 18 months to 4 years

Balanced characteristics:
- Responsible, reliable
- Balanced, effective willpower
- Good self esteem
- Able to feel your feelings
- Able to discern the difference between what you feel and what other people are feeling
- Confident
- Warm
- Relaxed

Physical malfunctions:
- Eating disorders
- Digestive disorders
- Liver, gallbladder, spleen or pancreas problems

- Hypoglycemia or diabetes
- Chronic fatigue
- Muscle spasms

Affirmations
- I honor who I am and who I have a right to be
- It is safe for me to feel my feelings
- I can do whatever I will to do
- I take pride in my work
- I keep my word
- I respect myself
- I know who I am
- I can say no when I need to

To heal wounds of your 3rd chakra:
- Protect your solar plexus by imagining a screen in front of it
- Visualize energy coming from the crown of your head and pushing out from your 3rd chakra like water pouring out of a fire hydrant
- Express your anger in appropriate ways, punch a pillow, roll up the windows of your car and yell
- Ask yourself how you are really feeling
- Take risks
- Deep relaxation, stress management
- Martial arts
- Learn to say no
- Develop your willpower
- Eat yellow fruits and vegetables
- Balance your blood sugar

Sound: Ram, E note

Yoga postures that benefit your 3rd chakra:
- Spinal twists, bow, wheel, bridge, seated boat, lying facing boat, reverse plank, breath of joy, warrior poses, sun salutes

4th Chakra, Anahata, Heart Chakra

Purpose: To give and receive love

Issues:
Love
- Balance
- Self-nurturing
- Relationships
- Devotion
- Reaching out and taking in
- Balance between the physical and spiritual
- Body-mind integration

If the 4th chakra is deficient:
- Withdrawn, cold, antisocial
- Judgmental
- Intolerant of self or others
- Depression
- Loneliness
- Fear of intimacy
- Lack of empathy
- Narcissism

If the 4th chakra is excessive:
- Codependent
- Demanding
- Clinging
- Jealousy
- Overly sacrificing
- Giving too much

Color: Green

Gland: Thymus

Developmental age: 4 to 7 years

Balanced characteristics:
- Compassionate
- Loving
- Empathetic
- Self loving
- Altruistic
- Peaceful
- Strong immune system
- Happy

Physical malfunctions:
- Heart problems
- Lung problems
- Immune deficiency
- Breathing difficulties
- Circulatory problems
- Tension between shoulder blades

Affirmations:
- I love myself unconditionally
- I am able to give and receive love
- I balance giving and receiving in my life
- I deserve to be loved
- There is an infinite supply of love in my life
- I am the place that love flows through
- I am loving to myself and others
- I love what I do
- I am surrounded by love and support

To heal wounds of your 4th chakra:
Carry your own baby picture
- Write yourself a love letter
- Eat green fruits and vegetables
- Create a spiritual family of friends who really love you
- Say I am sorry to someone you need to
- Adopt an animal from the pet rescue
- Write a gratitude list
- Work with your arms
- Hug and be hugged
- Forgive yourself and others
- Journal
- Breathing exercises
- Do what you love to do

Sound: Yam, F note

Yoga postures that benefit your 4th chakra:
- Backbends, fish, camel, bridge, wheel, cobra, child, upward facing dog, sage twist, triangle,

balancing half moon

5th Chakra, Vissudha, Throat Chakra

Purpose: Center for psychic communication

Issues:
- Communication
- Creativity
- Listening
- Finding one's own voice
- Resonation

If the 5th chakra is deficient:
- Fear of speaking your mind
- Small voice
- Tone deaf
- Shy, introverted
- Difficulty putting your feelings into words

If the 5th chakra is excessive:
- Talk too much
- Unable to listen or understand
- Gossiping
- Dominating voice
- You interrupt others

Color: Blue

Glands: Thyroid, parathyroid

Developmental age: 7 to 12 years

Balanced characteristics:
- Good listener
- Resonant voice
- Good sense of timing and rhythm
- Clear communication
- Creative

Physical malfunctions:
- Thyroid problems
- Disorders of neck, throat, jaw and ears
- Toxicity in the body
- Voice problems

Affirmations:
- I speak my truth with love and grace
- I express myself clearly
- I listen with my whole heart
- I allow my thoughts to flow
- I speak from my heart

To heal wounds of your 5th chakra:
Play a musical instrument
- Write letters that you later burn and release to the universe
- Practice silence
- Listen to music
- Sing, chant, tone
- Tell stories
- Write in a journal
- Laugh
- Express who you really are
- Eat blue fruits

Sound: Ham, G note

Yoga poses that heal your 5th chakra:
- Shoulderstand, fish, neck stretches, neck rolls, rabbit, plow, knee to ear pose

6th Chakra, Ajna, Third Eye Chakra

Purpose: Psychic vision

Issues:
- Vision
- Intuition
- Imagination
- Visualization
- Insight
- Dreams
- Visions

If your 6th chakra is deficient:
- Insensitivity
- Poor vision
- Poor memory
- Difficulty seeing the future or alternatives
- Lack of imagination
- Difficulty visualizing
- Can't remember dreams
- Denial—can't see what's really going on

If your 6th chakra is excessive:
- Hallucinations
- Obsessions
- Delusions
- Difficulty concentrating
- Nightmares

Color: Indigo, a blend of red and blue

Gland: Pituitary

Developmental age: Adolescence

Balanced characteristics:
- Intuitive
- Perceptive
- Good memory
- Imaginative
- Able to access and remember dreams
- Able to visualize
- Able to think symbolically

Physical malfunctions:
- Eye problems
- Headaches

Affirmations:
- It is safe for me to see the truth
- My life evolves with clarity
- I honor my psychic vision
- I can manifest my vision
- I am open to the wisdom within

- I imagine wonderful things for my life
- I like what I see

To heal wounds of your 6th chakra:
- Get enough natural sunlight
- Purchase a light therapy box
- Meditate
- Create visual art - paint, draw
- Meditate
- Visit art galleries
- Look at beautiful scenery
- Climb to the top of a mountain and enjoy the view
- Always look your best
- Get a makeover
- Surround yourself with beauty
- Use full spectrum lightbulbs
- Garden

Sound: Om, A note

Yoga postures that benefit 6th chakra:
- Meditation, lotus, yoga mudra, cow's head, dancer, spinal twists, plough, bridge, shoulderstand, eagle

7th chakra, Sahasrara, Crown Chakra

Purpose: Psychic knowing

Issues:
- Spirituality
- Connection to God
- Transcendence
- Belief systems
- Union
- Wisdom and mastery

If your 7th chakra is deficient:
- Depression
- Spiritual cynicism
- Learning difficulties
- Rigid belief systems
- Apathy

If your 7th chakra is excessive:
- Over intellectual
- Spiritual addiction
- Confusion
- Disassociation from the body

Color: Violet fading to white

Gland: Pineal

Developmental age: Early adulthood

Balanced characteristics:
- Spiritual outlook on life
- Able to learn easily
- Intelligent, thoughtful, aware
- Open minded
- Humble before the beauty and wonder of the universe

Physical malfunctions:
- Head injury
- Mental illness
- Coma
- Migraines
- Brain tumors
- Amnesia

Affirmations:
- I honor the divinity within me
- I am connected to God and all that is
- I am guided by my higher power
- I am guided by a higher wisdom
- I honor my knowing
- I follow my inner guidance
- Information I need comes to me whenever I need it
- I am a soul with a physical body
- I am passionate about my life
- I do the best I can
- I am open to new learning
- I accept all parts of myself
- I accept everything that happens in my life as a blessing from God

- I know and experience that I am blessed by God

To heal wounds of your 7th chakra:
- Read spiritual literature
- Attend church, synagogue, or meditate regularly
- Wear white clothing
- Connect your body, mind, and spirit
- Pray
- Attend programs of learning and study
- Listen to the silence
- Use "cancel that" for any negativity
- Practice watching your thoughts
- Talk to God
- Rest one day a week

Made in the USA
Lexington, KY
22 November 2019